DEEP TISSUE MASSAGE TREATMENT

SECOND EDITION

Jeffrey A. Simancek, BS, NCMT

Owner/Therapist—Wolf Tracks Massage Therapy
Irvine, California

ELSEVIER
MOSBY

3251 Riverport Lane
St. Louis, Missouri 63043

DEEP TISSUE MASSAGE TREATMENT, Second Edition

ISBN: 978-0-323-07759-0

Notices

Knowledge and best practice in this field are constantly changing. As new research and experience broaden our understanding, changes in research methods, professional practices, or medical treatment may become necessary.

Practitioners and researchers must always rely on their own experience and knowledge in evaluating and using any information, methods, compounds, or experiments described herein. In using such information or methods they should be mindful of their own safety and the safety of others, including parties for whom they have a professional responsibility.

With respect to any drug or pharmaceutical products identified, readers are advised to check the most current information provided (i) on procedures featured or (ii) by the manufacturer of each product to be administered, to verify the recommended dose or formula, the method and duration of administration, and contraindications. It is the responsibility of practitioners, relying on their own experience and knowledge of their patients, to make diagnoses, to determine dosages and the best treatment for each individual patient, and to take all appropriate safety precautions.

To the fullest extent of the law, neither the Publisher nor the authors, contributors, or editors, assume any liability for any injury and/or damage to persons or property as a matter of products liability, negligence or otherwise, or from any use or operation of any methods, products, instructions, or ideas contained in the material herein.

Library of Congress Cataloging-in-Publication Data

Simancek, Jeffrey A.
    Deep tissue massage treatment / Jeffrey A. Simancek. – 2nd ed.
        p. ; cm.
    Rev. ed. of: Deep tissue massage treatment / Enrique Fabian Fernandez. c2006
    Includes bibliographical references and index.
    ISBN 978-0-323-07759-0 (pbk. : alk. paper)
    I. Fernandez, Enrique Fabian. Deep tissue massage treatment. II. Title.
    [DNLM: 1. Massage–methods–Handbooks. WB 39]
    615.8'22–dc23
                                                                            2012004703

Vice President: Linda Duncan
Executive Content Strategist: Kellie White
Senior Content Development Specialist: Jennifer Watrous
Content Coordinator: Emily Thomson
Publishing Services Manager: Julie Eddy
Project Manager: Jan Waters
Design Direction: Amy Buxton

Printed in India

Last digit is the print number: 9 8 7 6 5 4 3

REVIEWERS

Debra S. Stell, MA, BA, LMT
National Training Director - Body Services
Elizabeth Arden Red Door Spas
Stamford, CT

Barbara G. White, LMT, MTI, NCTMB
Licensed Massage Therapist, Neuromuscular Therapist, Massage Instructor and
  Seminar Speaker
ABMP
Port Neches, Texas

PREFACE

"Skepticism is as much the result of knowledge, as knowledge is of skepticism. To be content with what we at present know, is, for the most part, to shut our ears against conviction; since, from the very gradual character of our education, we must continually forget, and emancipate ourselves from, knowledge previously acquired; we must set aside old notions and embrace fresh ones; and as we learn, we must be daily unlearning something which it has cost us no small labour and anxiety to acquire."

-Theodore Alois Buckley

According to the 2010 AMTA Industry Fact Sheet, 77 percent of massage therapists report offering deep tissue massage as one of the modalities they offer. Most schools have a portion of their curriculum dedicated to the application of deep tissue massage. This book was written to address the desire and need to better support the teaching and understanding of what deep tissue massage is and how to appropriately integrate it into the services massage therapists offer.

Deep Tissue Massage Treatment is comprised of two distinct and separate parts. The first four chapters are written to provide the reader with historical and theoretical backgrounds. It is necessary for the massage therapist to understand the how's and why's of application before the techniques can be applied in the most beneficial manner. The second part, which includes Chapters 5 through 10, reviews some of the basic anatomy of the body by region and some common pathological conditions experienced in each of these regions. Sample sequences are presented for a visual application of some of these techniques.

A few texts are available on the subject of deep tissue massage and many of these texts emphasize the techniques used. Few of these books emphasize the theoretical applications of these techniques. *Deep Tissue Massage Treatment* presents a review of the forces a massage therapist applies to the body, assessment approaches and a brief history on other modalities which are used to create a superior massage session for both the massage therapist and the client.

This edition has received several additions and updates. The theoretical and historical information in Chapter 1 offers a more detailed approach to the benefits and applications of deep tissue massage. The assessment section has more information and supportive documentation to aid you in the assessment of each client. The modalities presented in the first edition have been combined into Chapter 3 and updated with more information on each technique and approach to care. A chapter on proper tools and techniques (Chapter 4) has been added to help prevent stress and injury to the therapist. All the pathologic conditions presented in the first edition now include a brief background in the pathology and are sectioned off by body region rather than by condition. A brief overview of the anatomy is included to help you understand how the body works as a whole and may contribute to a particular condition. New images and videos on the Evolve site have been added to support each sequence in this book. Anatomical images have been used in each chapter to help visualize the information being presented in this book.

This book will be a key resource to have in your office, massage room or at home. In the appendix, you will find quick resource guides for common charting forms, terminology and trigger point referral patterns. Chapter 2 focuses on assessments and documentation for a deep tissue massage therapist and is accompanied by blank forms in the appendix for your use with clients. Chapter 3 provides historical and theoretical overviews of common modalities and techniques used during a deep tissue massage session. Proper use of your hands, elbows, forearms and fingers can be found in Chapter 4 to help prevent stress and injury to you as a therapist and aid in a long and rewarding career in the massage industry.

This edition includes multiple appendixes designed for your use. They contain blank intake forms, assessment forms and a variety of charting forms that can be copied for your use in the office. They also have a quick reference chart of common trigger points and pain referral patterns for a visual guide.

This text also comes with the Elsevier Evolve site as an ancillary at http://evolve.elsevier.com/Simancek/deeptissuemassage/. The site includes an instructor's manual, a 200-question ExamView test bank, an Image Collection, the appendixes, and downloadable forms. For convenience, all the videos on the pathologic conditions have been posted to the Evolve website for easy access from your home or office, making it easier to reference important material when you need to.

Deep tissue massage therapy is a diverse and functional approach to addressing the chronic short muscles of the body. Postural muscles are under a lot of stress and are working hard through the day. Alleviating the tension in these deeper tissues will provide your client with relief and comfort. When applied properly, deep tissue massage relieves stress, tension and pain from the receiver. Strong knowledge in anatomy, physiology and kinesiology is important to a successful massage session. Using the most appropriate hand position and technique for the body part you are working will save your body from stress and hard work. Work through the layers of the muscle, do not force the tissue, be patient and let the body soften and allow you access to the deeper structures. Utilize this book and continue to practice and fine-tune your techniques and you will take your clients to a new level of pain reduction and stress reduction.

ACKNOWLEDGMENTS

I would like to thank so many people for their support, suggestions, and words of encouragement. To my wife and son, there are no words that can truly express my appreciation for everything you have done for me and the support you have given me. For my parents, aunts, uncles, and cousins, thank you for your suggestions, conversations and, in some cases, debates, thank you.

A special thank you to Carol Lopresti who opened my eyes to the wonderful world of massage, to Ken for opening the door to education, and for all my mentors who have shared their knowledge of the industry with me.

None of this could have happened without the extremely talented team at Elsevier. Kelly Milford, Jennifer Watrous, Kellie White, Emily Thomson, Abby Hewitt, Lori Sypher, Jan Waters, as well as the video and photography staff – Jim Visser, Chuck LeRoi, and Chris Roider. Thank you to all for your help, support, patience, comments, and contributions without which this book would not have been created.

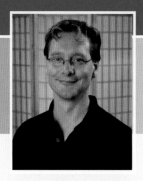

ABOUT THE AUTHOR

Jeffrey Simancek has been in the health and wellness industry for 20 years. He has worked as a personal trainer and managed health and fitness centers, practiced massage therapy as an independent contractor, taught massage therapy courses, and has written and managed curriculums for massage therapy. He has a Bachelor of Science in Health Science, with an emphasis in Exercise Science from Grand Valley State University. He is a NCBTMB certified Massage Therapist, California Certified Massage Therapist, and is a NCBTMB Approved Continuing Education Provider. He has worked in Physical Therapy Clinics, Fitness and Yoga centers, Chiropractic offices and still maintains his private practice and teaches for a local school.

CONTENTS

CONTENTS

DEEP TISSUE MASSAGE TREATMENT

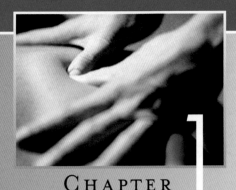

CHAPTER 1

THEORY

KEY TERMS

bend
compression
deep tissue
gravitational forces
homeostasis
mechanical forces
modalities
pain-spasm-pain cycle
shear
stress
stressor
tensile force
tension
torsion

OBJECTIVES

1. Discuss definitions of *deep tissue massage*.
2. Understand what is meant by *deep tissues*.
3. Explain the forces that act on the tissues of the body.
4. Understand how tension works.

Deep tissue massage therapy is one of the most frequently requested services in the massage profession. Many massage therapists recognize this and offer this modality. **Deep tissue** massage is commonly misunderstood and it can be unclear whether clients are requesting a deep tissue massage session or are asking for a massage with stronger pressure. Many clients often associate deep tissue massage with pain, hard or strong pressure, and often invasive massage techniques. Although there is a level of truth to this association, a good deep tissue session should not cause pain or discomfort. There may be a delayed onset of muscle soreness; however, any type of massage approach can cause this. Many schools often teach deep tissue massage as a technique that uses increased pressure to access the deeper layers of the tissues, often inadvertently overlooking the diverse applications of deep tissue massage techniques.

In this book we explore approaches to the applications and approaches to accessing the deeper tissues of the body. In Part 1, we explore the theoretical approaches like force, nature of tension, and pain and benefits of deep tissue massage.

We also look at the importance of postural, functional, and gait assessments as well as some of the common **modalities** that are important to deep tissue massage. Part 1 ends with an overview of the tools and techniques used during deep tissue sessions. Part 2 breaks the body down into smaller regions and addresses common pathologic conditions experienced in those regions for which a deep tissue approach may be beneficial.

THEORETICAL APPROACH

As a modality, deep tissue massage focuses on addressing the muscular complaints that are rooted in the deeper layers of the musculoskeletal system. Deep tissue massage should not be viewed as a separate modality, but rather as the use of several different techniques of therapeutic massage to enhance the overall outcome of the session. Deep tissue massage is a mindset, an intention, and an approach using the tools and talents possessed by a therapist to address specific musculoskeletal complaints (Figure 1-1).

Deep tissue massage is one of the most versatile and effective techniques for musculoskeletal complaints. It integrates techniques from Swedish Massage, Therapeutic Touch, Neuromuscular Techniques, Myofascial Techniques, and Structural Integration to address all levels of the body. A deep tissue session uses

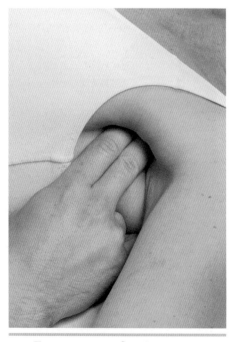

FIGURE 1-1 ■ Deep tissue massage.

techniques from these foundational approaches to work through the layers of the body as needed to reach the target muscle. Deep tissue integration is effective because it is an outcome-based approach and uses the techniques necessary to reach a desired outcome. Knowledge and understanding in anatomy, physiology, and kinesiology is extremely important in deep tissue approaches.

FORCES APPLIED TO THE BODY

Kinesiology and pathology are important tools to understand some of the causes for the muscular pain and holding patterns expressed by the client. Understanding the forces that play on the body helps in the application of the proper techniques to help with pain management and aid in the restoration of **homeostasis**. There are two primary classifications of forces that play on the body. These are *fields* and *mechanical forces*. Fields are forces like magnetic and electrical forces, which we have limited control over. **Mechanical forces** such as resistance and gravity are forces we have some control over. These forces can be the cause of the injury, but can also be applied to the body to remove the restrictions and tension that is causing the pain. Five main types of mechanical forces are applied to the body: compression, tension, torsion, shear, and bend.

COMPRESSION

Compression occurs when two or more structures are pushed together. This occurs with most massage strokes, but it also occurs in everyday life and injuries. Compression as a force can be beneficial or detrimental to the body (Figure 1-2).

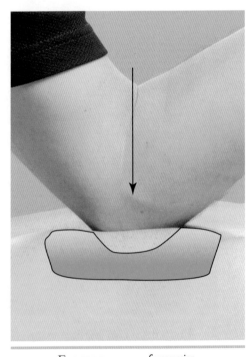

FIGURE 1-2 ■ Compression.

Many structures are susceptible to the effects of negative compressive forces. Nerves may become impinged between bone and muscle or compressed between muscles. The vertebrae are under constant compressive forces when standing and because of poor posture. Whether structures are pinched between bone and muscles, bone and bone, or by a narrowing of the passageways they travel through, the end result can be numbness and tingling or potential degenerative and compressive disorders.

Compression may be applied in beneficial ways as well. Ischemic compression is often applied to help dilate the vessels to encourage local circulation. Direct static pressure is used to help with muscle release and local congestion and is found in modalities like zone therapy, reflexology, trigger point therapy, shiatsu, and others.

TENSION

Although **tension** is often synonymous with **stress,** this is not the only manner in which it affects the body. Tensile forces are experienced throughout the day and in every activity. A **tensile force** is when the ends of the object are being pulled in the opposite direction from each other (Figure 1-3).

This is the force that is applied during any elongation or stretching motion. Injuries such as sprains and strains are examples of tensile forces applied to the body in a sudden or extreme manner. The sudden elongation or hyperextension of the area can result in ligamental, tendon, muscle, or bone damage.

When tension is applied properly, it can be used as a preventative, rehabilitative, or general health approach. When working the ends of the range of motion, we are applying tension to the muscle to encourage its elongation potential. Static stretching, postisometric relaxation, reciprocal inhibition, and proprioceptive neuromuscular facilitation are some techniques that use tensile forces to increase function and range of motion.

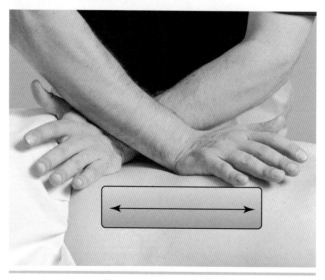

FIGURE 1-3 ■ Tension.

TORSION

Torsion is the application of a twisting or turning force to an object. This twisting force most often involves movement in one direction at one end of an object and stability or movement in the opposite direction at the other end (Figure 1-4*A*). During this movement both tensile and compressive forces act on a specific area at the same time (Figure 1-4*B*).

Twisting force applied to a structure that is not as pliable, such as a bone, may result in spiral fracture. If torsion is applied to a joint such as the knee, it may result in damage to the meniscus or tears to the ligaments.

When applied with appropriate force, torsion can be a beneficial technique. Many kneading techniques use torsion forces to help loosen and soften the muscle tissue.

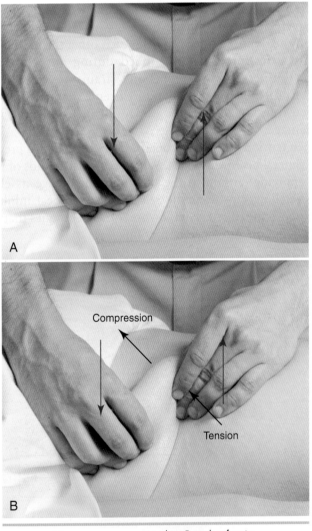

A

Compression

Tension

B

FIGURE 1-4 ■ **A** and **B,** Examples of torsion.

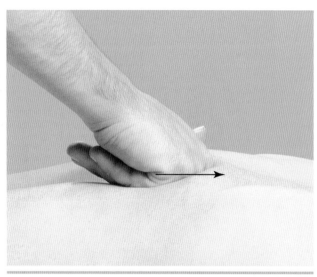

FIGURE 1-5 ■ Shear.

SHEAR

Shear forces are common throughout everyday activities. The act of squatting to pick up a box, walking downhill, and many sports involve shear forces. A shear force is when two structures slide across each other and create friction. This force, if repeated often, can result in adhesions or fibrosis within structures such as tendons (Figure 1-5).

Many common pathologic conditions result from repetitive shear forces such as tendonitis and inflammatory disorders. If shear force is applied suddenly and in excessive amounts, ligamental and joint tears may occur. Anterior cruciate ligament tear is an example of damage caused by shear force.

Massage therapists apply shear force in many of their techniques. Most gliding, stripping, and friction strokes use shear forces to help break adhesion and realign fibers. Depending on the depth of pressure and direction of application, shear forces can have a diverse array of effects.

BEND

Bending forces are also a result of compression and tension combined in one action. Bending involves an external force that is applied perpendicular to the axis of the object. Much like torsion, a compressive force is applied to one side of the object while the other side is exposed to tensile forces (Figure 1-6).

The main difference between bending and torsion is in the directions of the application of force. Bending is a linear force, whereas torsion is more of a rotational force. Many kneading techniques involve the application of bending because soft tissues are not as susceptible to the dangers of this force. Proprioceptors like Golgi tendon organs and muscle spindle cells are receptive to this force.

Bending forces are more dangerous to the more dense structures like bone. Many causes of bone breaking are attributed to a bending force. Many lateral and medial collateral ligament tears and ruptures are attributed to bending and shear forces combined.

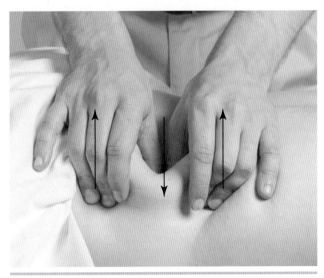

FIGURE 1-6 ▪ Bend.

THE NATURE OF TENSION AND DISCOMFORT

To better assess and treat musculoskeletal pain, there must be an understanding of where the discomfort and pain originate from. Many of the complaints that clients experience originate from the deeper musculature that are primarily used for stabilization and posture. Our daily activities and lifestyles tend to put demand on our musculoskeletal system, which often leads to chronic patterns of tension and stress. Workers who sit at a desk all day often experience shortening and tightening of the hip flexors, mill workers experience repetitive stress to the shoulder, and tennis players experience repetitive stress to their elbows.

Naturally occurring forces like gravity create stress and tension throughout the body, especially on the joints and musculature that support and stabilize the body. Sitting in front of a computer with one's head leaning forward and increased kyphotic curvature forces the deep erectors of the spine to work harder to maintain the position and compensate the load being applied to the body (Figure 1-7*A*). The same can be seen with people who wear backpacks over one shoulder or women carrying heavy, large purses (Figure 1-7*B & C*). These changes in position are due to the **gravitational forces** on the body and the muscular compensation to maintain balance. Prolonged exposure to these positions trains the deep postural muscles to be hypertonic.

Another cause of muscular tension results from chronically contracted muscles and the neurologic patterns that they create. Constant contraction or repetitive movements result in shortened muscles, which can lead to pain and restricted motions, and can create postural holding patterns. These neurologic and muscular changes are a natural defense mechanism of the body to defend itself from further injury and perceived threats. As muscle tension builds, pain and stiffness increases. With this increase, people stop moving the area or compensate to try to stop the pain. This process is often referred to as the **pain-spasm-pain cycle.** The lack of movement decreases the circulation to that area, which affects the transportation of nutrients and removal of waste products, which may delay the healing process.

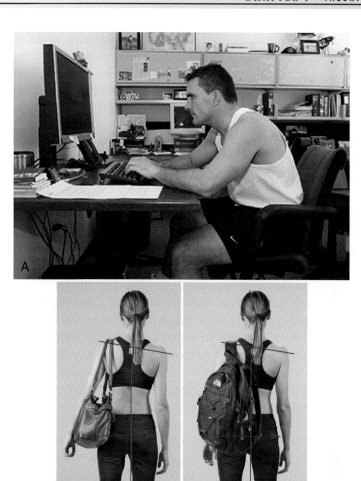

FIGURE 1-7 ■ **A-C,** Compensation patterns.

Life or emotional **stressors** are often involved in the chronic holding patterns, resulting in tension that clients experience. Stress reduction is a key focus of most massage therapy sessions and one of the leading reasons clients come through the door. Stress is the result of any internal or external stimulus that affects the homeostasis of the body, including the physical, physiologic, and emotional states. Whether the stressors are beneficial or not, these physiologic responses are complex chemical reactions that occur in the body. Common sources of stress can come from injuries and diseases, diet and nutrition, environment and pollution, and self-esteem and emotions.

Stress response systems, such as an increase in adrenaline prior to and during a sporting event, are beneficial to the body. However, chronic or sustained stressors that fatigue the body and impair function can result in damage and tension. Simply put, certain stressors can literally make people sick. These negative effects of stress often appear as shortness of breath, heart palpitations, insomnia, and gastrointestinal disturbances, not to mention the muscular soreness and increased potential for panic attacks and anxiety disorders.

CAUTION!

Working with emotional states is not a primary focus of therapeutic massage. Massage may result in emotional releases and clients should be referred when necessary to appropriate professionals.

EMOTIONS AND DEEP TISSUE MASSAGE

Muscular pain can present itself in holding patterns that have been caused by physical and psychological stressors. Psychologist Wilhelm Reich used the term *armoring* when he referred to the psychological stresses that become locked in muscular tension. Many massage therapists call these *emotional knots, stress knots,* or *trigger points.* Clients have the tendency to name them things like *"work, mother, kids,"* and so on. Regardless of what they are called, these areas may be caused by deep-seated emotions that have caused protective postures or armoring points. Massage therapy sessions may release this tension as well as the emotions, often referred to as an *emotional release.*

Working on a client who experiences an emotional release can make some therapists and clients uncomfortable. Every therapist should recognize the signs of an emotional release and how to approach the client during a release. Emotional releases can take many forms such as crying, laughing, anger, irritation, and even a feeling of relief. Every client reacts in a different manner. Some physical signs that an emotional release may occur or is occurring are changes in breathing patterns or body temperature, which is affected by blood flow to the skin. Some clients may start to fidget and rapid eye movements may occur. A distracted expression or a clench of the jaw or tight facial muscles may be due to the client feeling uncomfortable in letting go or trying to stop from crying. Showing signs of emotional vulnerability or crying in front of people may cause the client to tense up.

When an emotional release occurs, it is important that the therapist makes the client feel safe, secure, and comfortable. If the client is crying, offer her or him a tissue and a glass of water. Reassure the client that the emotional release may be beneficial and can be common in deep tissue massage. Reassure clients that the session is for them; if necessary they may stop the massage and take a moment for themselves.

APPROACH TO DEEP TISSUE MASSAGE

Some key approaches need to be followed when performing deep tissue massage techniques. Always be respectful of the client and his or her needs. Do not overstep the boundaries that you have set with your client. Remind the client that he or she is in control of the session. Be attentive to the subtle changes in body language; you may be using too much pressure or at a tender area where the client is more sensitive.

Never force the tissue. Move slowly as you go deeper in the layers of tissues. The deeper the tissue is, the slower the movement needs to be. Remember that the body needs to accept you into that level. Forcing tissues to move can increase the chance

Box 1-1 BENEFITS OF DEEP TISSUE MASSAGE

- Decrease muscular soreness.
- Increase mobility.
- Aid in improving posture.
- Release chronic tension.
- Increase oxygenation and nutrition to muscles.
- Relieve tension.
- Help address trigger points.
- Stretch muscles and fascia.
- Help address muscular imbalances.

of soreness. Delayed-onset soreness is often expected with deep tissue massage, but bruising or immense pain should not occur. Overworking a client and causing pain is crossing a line, which can discourage the client and prevent him or her from rescheduling. Deep tissue therapists work in areas and with techniques that can push the client's pain threshold; however, the intention is not to cause pain.

BENEFITS OF DEEP TISSUE MASSAGE

One of the goals of deep tissue massage is to elongate chronically shortened muscles and release muscular tension. This is to help the body return to a state of homeostasis. Other benefits for deep tissue massage are decreasing muscular tension and increasing mobility at the joints. Improvements in body posture may occur because the therapist addresses the tension and issues at a deeper layer of tissues and the postural muscles. Deep tissue techniques are built on many different modalities of massage, which aid in the relief of trigger points and muscular imbalances. Deep tissue massage also helps with circulation and increases oxygenation and nutrition to the cells and tissues (Box 1-1).

SUMMARY

There are several reasons why therapists need to understand the effects of various forms of tension on the body. Depending on the structure, muscle, or nerves that are affected by these forces, different outcomes will be experienced. When working with clients there are two important concepts to remember. One is that the pain that the client is experiencing is not always from a recent activity or injury. Compensation patterns, protective measures, and emotional tensions may create long-term muscular discomfort. Most musculoskeletal complaints are due to years of wear and tear, holding patterns, and abuse to the body. The other concept to remember is that the pain the clients feel is not always experienced at the site where the injury occurred. For example, neck pain is often a result of an imbalance in the hips or a curvature in the spine.

Deep tissue massage is a versatile and effective approach that affects the deeper layers of muscles and fascia. These techniques require advanced understanding of anatomy, physiology, kinesiology, and the effects of stress. Deep tissue massage helps with chronic muscular pain and rehabilitation and holding patterns that are caused by everyday life and tension. Deep tissue is a combination of a variety of techniques to help restore and maintain homeostasis.

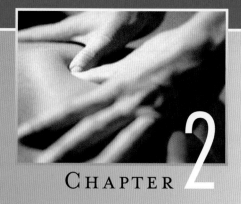

CHAPTER 2

ASSESSMENT

KEY TERMS

anterior tilt
assessment
closed kinematic chains
compensation patterns
hyperkyphosis
hyperlordosis
kinematics
kinetic chain
lower crossed syndrome
normal posture
objective
open kinematic chains
plan
postural assessment
posture
primary postural distortion
scoliosis
secondary postural distortion
subjective
upper crossed syndrome

OBJECTIVES

1 Explain the importance of assessment for the massage therapist.
2 Understand the role documentation has in massage sessions.
3 Be knowledgeable and apply skills in postural assessments.
4 Recognize postural deviations.
5 Understand postural distortion patterns.

ASSESSMENTS

As therapists know, one of the most important components of a session is the **assessment**. A good assessment should include a thorough interview. This helps guide the therapist toward the best approach for that individual. This interview should include questioning on the client's employment and job duties, and whether the pain is work related. It is also important to know if there have been other accidents or injuries in the past that may contribute to this discomfort. This is also a good time to get more clarity on the type of pain the client is experiencing. Pain sensations are unique and can help guide the therapist to the type of injury causing the pain.

Documentation is a crucial part of the assessment process. Documenting all findings, **subjective** and **objective**, before and after the session will demonstrate whether the approach to care is working. When working with other parties such as other therapists, doctors, insurance companies, and so on, documenting what approach was taken and what changes have occurred is beneficial to all. The "subjective, objective, assessment, and plan," or SOAP note is a universal way of tracking progress over sessions. It is used by most medical facilities and it is suggested that therapists use this method for documentation. Other key forms to use are client histories, health histories, evaluations, body maps, and an initial consultation for first-time clients. Sample forms can be found in the appendix.

With all assessments, it is important to document the details of the tests performed. Be specific with the notes so the test can be repeated in the future. The position, type of test, joint, and action should be clearly noted. Identify and rate any deviations from normal as well as potential causes for any limitations. These details can be recorded during an initial body assessment and reassessments.

The interview and health intake process helps clarify the client's medical history. Medical histories are important to determine whether massage is contraindicated for that client. It is also important to learn about any medications the client might be taking. Many medications can interfere with the session or at least alter the responses the therapist receives. General pain killers, for example, if taken before the session, may numb the client's pain sensations, which could result in inaccurate feedback. This could cause the therapist to use more pressure, which may do more damage than good. This is a big concern when using deep tissue massage.

Being thorough with your interview helps create an ideal treatment **plan** for the future. If the process of designing a treatment plan is seen as solving a puzzle, the interview process builds the border of the puzzle. Having an understanding of what has been going on with the client and what he or she is currently feeling will be helpful in focusing the attention of the therapist during the physical part of the assessment.

Experts suggest using a separate page specifically for the initial body assessment. This allows the therapist to complete a thorough assessment that can be referred to and compared with during future sessions. Forms should document all assessment methods such as postural assessment, gait assessment, and functional assessment.

POSTURAL ASSESSMENT

The postural assessment is a starting place for most massage therapists. Be cautious when performing a postural assessment. People automatically alter their **normal** standing position when the topic of **posture** is approached. During a **postural assessment**, the client needs to be in a natural, relaxed standing position. If it is necessary, have your client march in place for 30 seconds to 1 minute. Pay attention to the motion of the knees and hips. Be sure to have the client "pump" his or her arms during this motion; this can also be used as one of the functional assessments. Stop the motion and have the client stand in place without making any compensation.

Now the therapist can document head position, shoulder level, hips, knees, and ankles. Take a superficial glance at first, noting things like an asymmetrical stance, contours of the body, and body type. From the anterior view, look for the head position: are the mastoid processes even and balanced? Draw a mental line from acromion process to acromion process: are the shoulders level with each other? Look at the iliac crests and the anterior superior iliac spines: do they appear even? Also look at the head of the fibulas and the malleoli: are they even with each other? If necessary, palpate the structures to confirm your assessment (Figure 2-1).

From the lateral view the therapist should look for alignment of the body. Imagine a line perpendicular to the ground, or use a plumb line to assess the posture. This line should go through the external auditory meatus, acromioclavicular joint, greater trochanter, fibular head, and just anterior to the lateral malleolus (Figure 2-2). It is common to see **upper crossed syndromes** and **lower crossed syndromes** from this view. Understanding these crossed patterns and applying them throughout the body will help the therapist identify possible areas of weak muscles or hypertonic muscles.

Recognizing upper and lower crossed syndromes can help guide the therapist to an appropriate technique or approach. The upper crossed syndrome presents itself with a protracted shoulder girdle often caused by tightness in the pectorals and the posterior neck muscles. Hypertonicity in these muscles is compensated by weak anterior neck and lower trapezius muscles. The lower crossed syndrome is also prominent from a lateral view. This shows tight hip flexors and low back muscles, and weak abdominals and gluteals. The pelvis appears to tilt forward, often referred to as an anterior tilt (Figure 2-3).

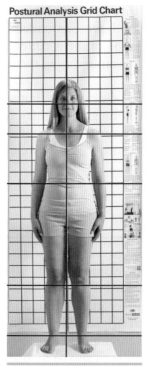

FIGURE 2-1 ■ Anterior postural assessment.

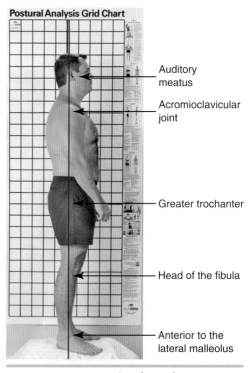

FIGURE 2-2 ■ Lateral postural assessment.

Auditory meatus

Acromioclavicular joint

Greater trochanter

Head of the fibula

Anterior to the lateral malleolus

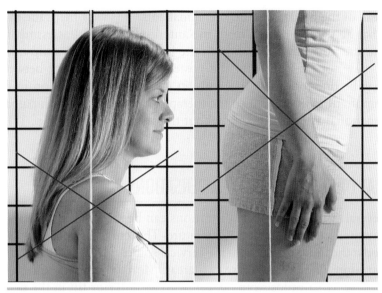

FIGURE 2-3 ■ Upper and lower crossed syndromes.

As with the other postural assessments, the therapist should look for symmetry of the contours of the back and alignment of the spine. This can be completed using a plumb line or an imaginary line perpendicular to the ground. Starting from the top down, look for the symmetry of the mastoid processes, acromion processes, inferior angle of the scapula, iliac crest, posterior superior iliac spine,

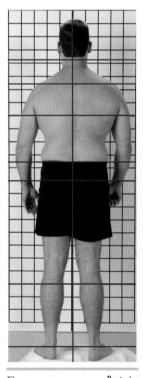

FIGURE 2-4 ■ Posterior postural assessment.

head of the fibula, and the lateral malleoli. This view helps the therapist confirm what he or she noticed from the anterior and lateral assessments. Although in the anterior view a deviation in the hips may look like a hip hike, or elevation, it may not be seen from the posterior. This inaccuracy between assessments may be due to a rotation versus an elevation or depression in the hip. This is important to document so the therapist can follow up with palpation and other functional assessments throughout the session (Figure 2-4, p. 15).

POSTURAL DISTORTIONS AND COMPENSATIONS

Several common postural distortions can be seen in the body. *Lordosis* refers to a natural ventral or anterior curvature. This curvature occurs in two areas of the body: the lumbar spine and the cervical spine. A **hyperlordosis** is an accentuated curvature of either of these two areas. More commonly known as *sway back,* a lumbar hyperlordosis can be seen with an **anterior tilt** in the pelvis and is often caused by tight low back and psoas major muscles. *Kyphosis* refers to the dorsal or posterior curvature seen in the thoracic vertebrae. **Hyperkyphosis**, often known as *humpback,* is often seen in those who have a forward head position. Another spinal curvature is known as **scoliosis**, which is a lateral curvature of the spine. Any of these curvatures may be the result of structural or functional disorders. Tight muscles, joint displacement, structural defects, and genetic disorders play a role in abnormal curvatures of the spine (Figure 2-5).

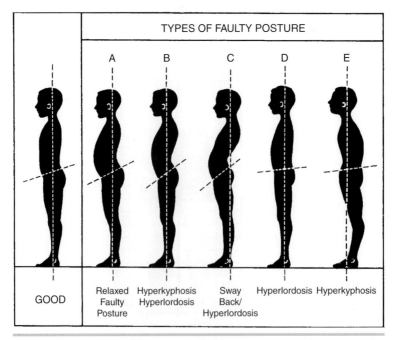

FIGURE 2-5 ■ Postural distortions. (Modified from McMorris RO: Faulty postures, *Pediatr Clin North Am* 8:217, 1961.)

With an understanding of the common postural distortions, the therapist can go into more depth with the muscular imbalances caused by improper posture. As stated earlier, the cause of the client's complaint often is not in the area where the complaint is felt. Muscular imbalances can create postural deviations that can result in impingements and compression discomforts. These imbalances end up causing other parts of the body to compensate to maintain balance. A client may show an elevated left shoulder, which results in the complaint of right shoulder pain. During the postural assessment the therapist may notice that the client overpronates the left foot while standing in a static stance. This shift in structural alignment causes the left hip to drop a little, which also drops the right shoulder, elevating the left. Another compensation that the body may undergo to maintain the shoulder is to create a lateral curvature in the spine (Figure 2-6).

A postural distortion pattern is a set of interrelated distortions within the body. There are two levels to these distortions, the primary and secondary. The **primary postural distortion** is due to problems in a specific area of the body. The **secondary postural distortion** can be found in another area of the body, often away from the primary. This secondary distortion is often caused by the primary distortion. Although it is beneficial to work the secondary distortion pattern, it is important to remember that it is not the source of the pain. Addressing the needs of the secondary pain will provide temporary relief of pain, but it will not address

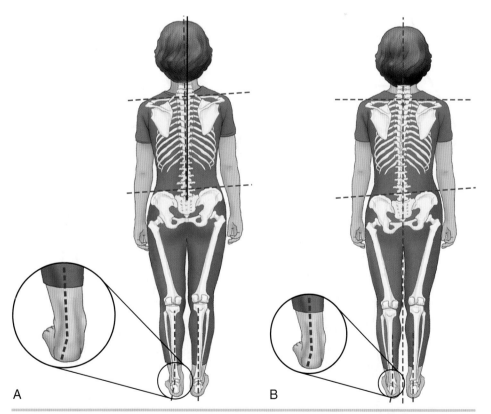

A   B

FIGURE 2-6 ■ **A** and **B**, Left foot compensations. (From Muscolino JE: *Kinesiology: the skeletal system and muscle function,* ed 2, St Louis, 2011, Mosby.)

the primary distortion that initiated the pain. Working through each distortion will help lead the therapist to the primary cause. This may not be revealed in one session, but can take several sessions to discover.

When the body becomes out of balance from the proper posture, the muscles become engaged to maintain the new posture. When the body makes adjustments to maintain its balance and stability, it is called a **compensation pattern**. As an example, if a person's right leg is shorter than the left, a shift in the left knee alignment would be visible when the client is in a standing position. This would then cause the left hip to drop, which in turn would create a lateral curvature, which would be seen as a right depressed shoulder and lateral flexed neck to the left. Because of the forces being pulled to maintain an upright position, some muscles become tight and short, whereas others are in a constant state of elongation (Figure 2-7).

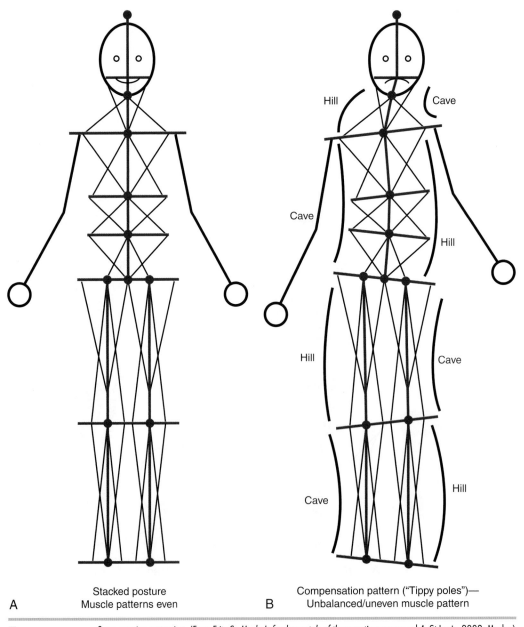

A   Stacked posture
Muscle patterns even

B   Compensation pattern ("Tippy poles")—
Unbalanced/uneven muscle pattern

FIGURE 2-7 ■ Compensation patterning. (From Fritz S: *Mosby's fundamentals of therapeutic massage,* ed 4, St Louis, 2009, Mosby.)

Compensation is the automatic response the body makes to maintain balance to the internal or external environment. A deviation from anatomic posture results in a shift or change in body alignment and muscle tone to keep the body erect and balanced. Within the musculoskeletal system, this can be observed not only with the posture, but with the joint motion as well. If a particular joint is hypermobile, it can become weak and unstable. This instability may cause other joints to become less mobile to compensate for this weakness. This weakness can also result in local muscle contractions and tension to help protect the joint. This tightness in the musculature can be overdone, resulting in a hypomobile joint. The balance is needed for the body to operate optimally.

GAIT CYCLE

Gait is defined as the process of loading and unloading weight in the legs during the act of motion. Your gait is the way you walk, jog, or run, and can vary based on terrain, speed, and other factors. It is a multifaceted process that requires many muscles to engage. A multitude of processes are working during the "simple" act of walking. Propulsive forces are created by the muscle contractions, equilibrium is constantly changing with the shift in the center of gravity, proprioceptors are coordinating to help control the movement of the limbs and joint positioning, and there is a collection of several sensory stimuli from all senses to move fluidly and rhythmically.

The gait cycle is a series of movements that starts with the heel strike and continues to the next heel strike of the same foot used to start the motion. One cycle is the equivalent to one stride or two steps. There are two phases in this cyclic movement pattern, each with specific movements within each phase. The stance phase starts this motion with the initial heel strike. This is the moment when the heel of the foot makes contact with the ground. Flat-foot starts when the weight shifts forward and is displaced across the plantar surface of the foot. This momentum continues to propel us forward, where we reach the midstance stage. This is where weight is distributed over one leg and the greater trochanter of the femur is directly over the middle of the foot. As weight continues to shift forward, the heel starts to come up off the ground. This is the heel-off stage, which leads into the toe-off stage, which marks the end of the stance phase of walking (Figure 2-8).

The swing phase starts at the toe-off stage. Once the foot leaves the ground, it moves through the early, mid, and late parts of the swing. Approximately 60% of the gait cycle is spent in the stance phase for each lower extremity. Many muscles and motions are executed during a gait cycle. The hip flexors contract to aid in the swing phase and the hip extensors eccentrically contract to control the momentum created during the swing. The hip abductors play several roles during the gait, especially stabilizing and maintaining level hips. The hip adductors isometrically contract to stabilize the hips during the heel strike and contract to aid in flexion just after toe-off. The rotators of the hip are primarily active during the stance phase to stabilize the hip joint. The extensors of the knees are working hard at the end of the swing phase to prepare for the heel strike and are also needed during the beginning of the stance phase to stabilize the knee for the weight transfer. The flexors, on the other hand, contract to slow the extension of the knee to prepare for the heel strike, stabilize and protect the knee joint during the heel strike, and contract to prevent the foot from dragging during the swing phase (Figure 2-9).

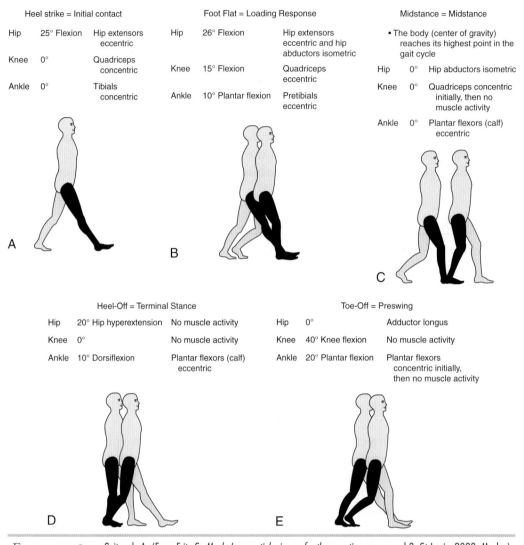

Heel strike = Initial contact

Hip	25° Flexion	Hip extensors eccentric
Knee	0°	Quadriceps concentric
Ankle	0°	Tibials concentric

Foot Flat = Loading Response

Hip	26° Flexion	Hip extensors eccentric and hip abductors isometric
Knee	15° Flexion	Quadriceps eccentric
Ankle	10° Plantar flexion	Pretibials eccentric

Midstance = Midstance

• The body (center of gravity) reaches its highest point in the gait cycle

Hip	0°	Hip abductors isometric
Knee	0°	Quadriceps concentric initially, then no muscle activity
Ankle	0°	Plantar flexors (calf) eccentric

A

B

C

Heel-Off = Terminal Stance

Hip	20° Hip hyperextension	No muscle activity
Knee	0°	No muscle activity
Ankle	10° Dorsiflexion	Plantar flexors (calf) eccentric

Toe-Off = Preswing

Hip	0°	Adductor longus
Knee	40° Knee flexion	No muscle activity
Ankle	20° Plantar flexion	Plantar flexors concentric initially, then no muscle activity

D

E

FIGURE 2-8 ■ Gait cycle A. (From Fritz S: *Mosby's essential sciences for therapeutic massage,* ed 3, St Louis, 2009, Mosby.)

GAIT ANALYSIS

Gait analysis is a way to assess the dynamic posture and coordination during movement. This analysis is a means to evaluate, record, and make any necessary corrections for a smooth gait. During this analysis the therapist needs to note the minor shifts in movement such as rotations and tilts or knee movement and foot placement. These movements can help lead the therapist to potential issues with flexibility and muscle strength. Identifying hypermobile or hypomobile movements at the joints, whether or not the movement varies from side to side, can help identify proprioceptor and neuromuscular concerns. Assessing any deviations or inconsistencies can be a clue to potential restrictions.

Be aware of your surroundings when performing a gait assessment. The client will become more conscious of his or her movements when you ask your

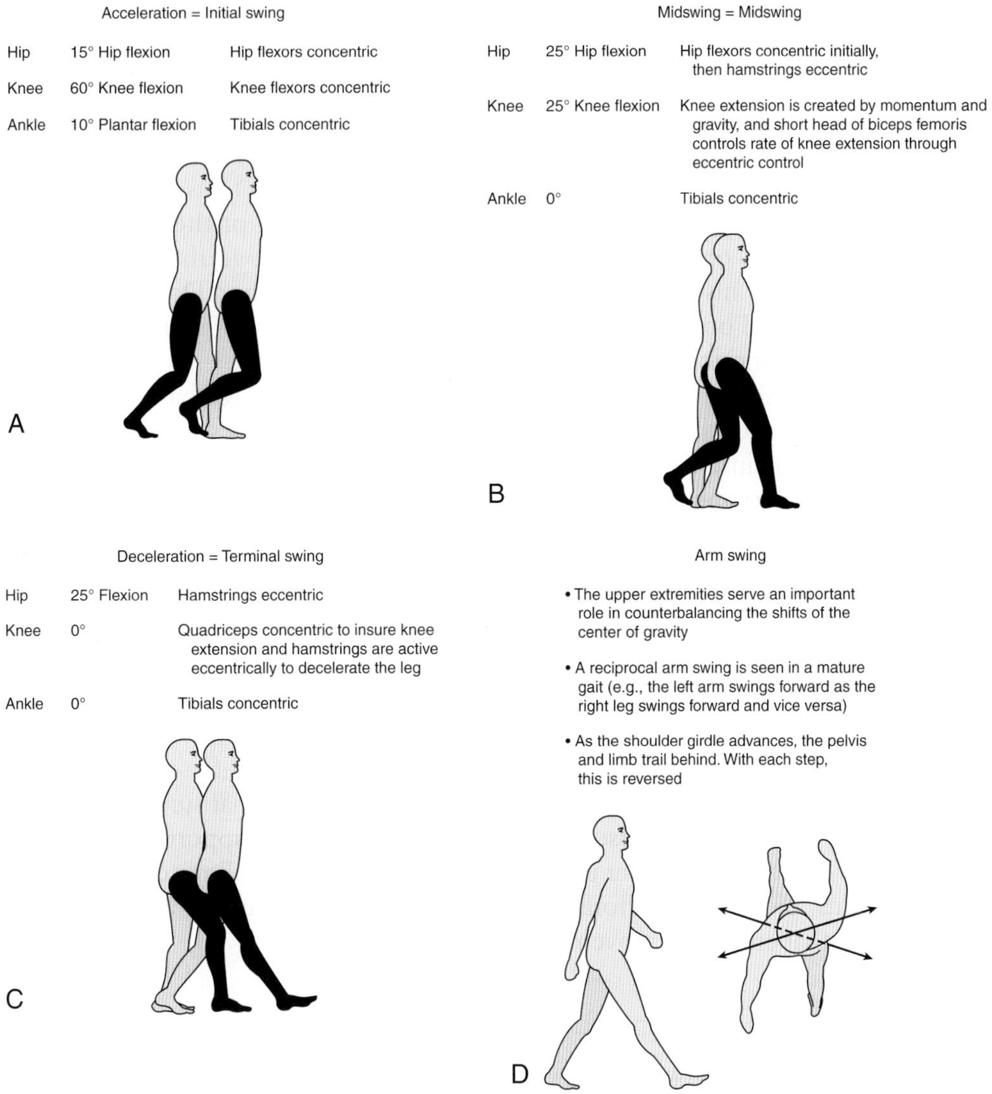

Acceleration = Initial swing

Hip	15° Hip flexion	Hip flexors concentric
Knee	60° Knee flexion	Knee flexors concentric
Ankle	10° Plantar flexion	Tibials concentric

A

Midswing = Midswing

Hip	25° Hip flexion	Hip flexors concentric initially, then hamstrings eccentric
Knee	25° Knee flexion	Knee extension is created by momentum and gravity, and short head of biceps femoris controls rate of knee extension through eccentric control
Ankle	0°	Tibials concentric

B

Deceleration = Terminal swing

Hip	25° Flexion	Hamstrings eccentric
Knee	0°	Quadriceps concentric to insure knee extension and hamstrings are active eccentrically to decelerate the leg
Ankle	0°	Tibials concentric

C

Arm swing

- The upper extremities serve an important role in counterbalancing the shifts of the center of gravity

- A reciprocal arm swing is seen in a mature gait (e.g., the left arm swings forward as the right leg swings forward and vice versa)

- As the shoulder girdle advances, the pelvis and limb trail behind. With each step, this is reversed

D

FIGURE 2-9 ■ Gait cycle B. (From Fritz S: *Mosby's essential sciences for therapeutic massage*, ed 3, St Louis, 2009, Mosby.)

client to walk for you. This altered motion caused by the client's awareness of being assessed may create false information. One recommendation is to have the client do some of the other assessments first and use the gait to fine tune your assessment. You can also observe your client while he or she is walking into your massage space, or as you guide him or her to your table.

Gait and posture may be affected by a number of factors that should be included in your findings. Structural deformations, wear and tear, previous injuries, and other findings can affect the way the body moves and the fluidity of the gait. The client's age, height, gender, and total body weight are all variables that also lead to understanding where the pain and dysfunctions originate.

FUNCTIONAL ASSESSMENTS

Functional assessments are methods that assess the body during movements. Range-of-motion (ROM) movements take the body through different movements and positions in which the therapist can assess the quality of the movement. The first focal point during ROM exercises is to assess the freedom of the movement. Have the client move through some of the basic activities he or she does on a daily basis, or have an athlete move through the basic movements of his or her sport. How fluid is the motion? Does it appear to be symmetrical on both sides? Are there obvious restrictions that show themselves in the motion?

A massage therapist should possess a strong knowledge base in anatomy, physiology, and kinesiology. Being skilled in biomechanics, open and closed kinematic chains, and ROM for the body are important in understanding functional assessments.

KINETIC CHAIN

A **kinetic chain** is defined as an "integrated functional unit." This usually consists of bones, joints, ligaments, tendons, muscle, fascia, and nerves. Each kinetic unit works interdependently to allow for structural and functional efficiency. Every movement consists of a complex compilation of acceleration, stabilization, and deceleration. Kinetic chains can be broken down into two different components to create a motion. The inner unit consists of the muscles that surround the joint that are moving. The muscles in this unit function to support, stabilize, and protect the joint. The outer unit consists of more superficial muscles such as the trapezius, bicep, and pectoralis major muscles. These muscles are the primary movers that create the movement at the joint.

KINEMATIC CHAIN

Kinematics is the study of how kinetic chains work together to create motion. A kinematic chain describes the association between joints as they operate in relation to each other. There are two types of kinematic chains: the closed chain and the open chain. Understanding how the joints work together can help the therapist identify the root of the client's complaint. For example, a client may complain about an upper trapezius pain; the root of the problem may be found in unbalanced hips, which has led to a lateral curvature in the spine, which could result in hypertonic muscle in the cervical area.

When assessing motion during certain movements in which more than one joint often moves, understanding how these joints work together to allow the motion to occur can help the therapist practice smarter with quicker results.

Closed Kinematic Chain

When the motion of one joint directly affects motion at another joint, it is considered a **closed kinematic chain**. To visualize this, picture a person squatting down to pick up a heavy box. The feet are solid on the ground, locking the position of the foot. The person, with correct body mechanics, bends his or her knees to reach the box. As the person gets lower, both the ankles and the hips must change their angles to allow motion to occur. These joint movements are linked together and can be predicted based on the movements necessary to perform the action.

Looking at these movements allows the therapist to note any kind of compensation that may need to be made because of a limiting factor, injury, or pain. Ideally, in the squatting motion, the back should remain straight and hips, knees, and ankles should travel along the same plane. If there is a restriction in the knee, the hip, or the ankle, the body will make a minor adjustment to allow the motion to occur. If the medial aspect of the knee is sore it may pry outward, causing the toes to turn out during the motion.

Open Kinematic Chain

Open kinematic chains are noted at the ends of the limbs or at the joint where it is free to move without causing motion at another joint. This can be easily observed by sitting in a chair and extending the knee. When a person is sitting and is asked to tighten the quadriceps to extend his or her knee, the only joint that is moving is the knee joint. Motion of the ankle and hip do not need to change their angles to allow knee extension to occur.

The open chain allows joints to function independently from each other. The joints above and below the moving joint do not need to compensate and their motions are not predictable. These joints have freedom to move or stabilize the joint without affecting the action of the other. Open chains can be beneficial to help pinpoint pain, discomfort, and potential injuries or restrictions. Open kinematic chains do not represent most motions in the activities of daily living.

KINETIC CHAIN PROTOCOL

Assessing gross movements gives the therapist a better idea of location and restrictions within a system. It is important to know which movements cause pain because of the restrictions or if the restrictions are due to a postural distortion of some form. These movements also narrow down the regions of the body to explore when there is a generalized complaint of pain.

During client movements, pay attention to the compensatory patterns of the body. Have the client march in place, and observe the right arm moving with the left leg. As the right arm reaches for the sky, the lower body must adjust to stack the joints and maintain balance. Just like the upper and lower crossed syndromes addressed earlier, compensations are made throughout the body. The right shoulder and left hip are connected through muscular and fascial chains. Visualizing the body in key body balancing points can help identify these compensation patterns. After identifying these segments, the therapist can start to assess the segments above, below, and opposite the area of complaint. This helps to identify the compensation patterns created and guides the therapist to the root of the complaint (Figure 2-10).

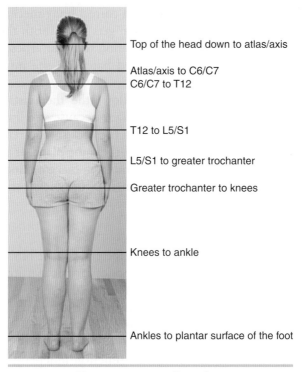

Top of the head down to atlas/axis

Atlas/axis to C6/C7

C6/C7 to T12

T12 to L5/S1

L5/S1 to greater trochanter

Greater trochanter to knees

Knees to ankle

Ankles to plantar surface of the foot

FIGURE 2-10 ■ Kinetic chain.

RANGE OF MOTION

ROM has benefits as both a technique as well as an assessment tool. By definition, ROM is the amount and type of motion available at a particular joint. ROM is usually categorized into two types of motion: anatomic and physiologic. Anatomic ROM is the normal amount of motion available at a specific location. Physiologic ROM is the amount of motion available as a result of general wear and tear patterns, and structural or neurologic limitations. The joint capsule, bone structures, muscle bulk, and ligaments often affect the amount of motion available. This motion is usually less than the anatomic ROM (Table 2-1).

The way ROM exercises or techniques are applied can help identify which type of structure or tissue may be restricted or injured. The posture and gait analysis help identify imbalances in the body. The functional analysis uses active ROM to assess muscular control and motions. It allows the therapist to see the quality and quantity of motion through a set motion. These should be performed on both sides, with the unaffected side first to assess any limitations.

Passive ROM can be used to assess the stability of the joints and ability of the antagonist muscles to elongate. Using passive motion or therapist-controlled motion allows the therapist to focus on the quality of the joint structure and ligaments. Taking the client's affected joint through its natural ROM should not cause pain within its structures. Any pain experienced during its range or failure

Table 2-1 RANGE OF MOTION

Neck flexion	50 degrees
Neck extension	60 degrees
Neck lateral flexion	45 degrees
Neck rotation	80 degrees
Back flexion	90 degrees
Shoulder flexion	150 degrees
Shoulder extension	50 degrees
Shoulder abduction	150 degrees
Shoulder adduction	30 degrees
Elbow flexion	150 degrees
Elbow extension	0 degrees
Forearm pronation	80 degrees
Forearm supination	80 degrees
Wrist flexion	60 degrees
Wrist extension	60 degrees
Radial deviation	20 degrees
Ulnar deviation	30 degrees
Back extension	25 degrees
Back lateral flexion	25 degrees
Hip flexion	100 degrees
Hip extension	20 degrees
Hip adduction	20 degrees
Hip abduction	40 degrees
Knee flexion	150 degrees
Knee extension	0 degrees
Plantar flexion	40 degrees
Dorsiflexion	20 degrees
Ankle inversion	30 degrees
Ankle eversion	20 degrees

Measurements based on goniometric readings

of the joint to reach the full range is a clue to a structural, neurologic, or muscular injury or dysfunction.

Resisted ROM engages the musculature that surrounds the joint. This stimulus to the muscles allows the therapist to assess the quality of the muscles and tendons of that joint. It is important to apply a counterforce against the path of motion, holding for approximately 8-10 second intervals along the way. Support the joints and control the path of motion to isolate specific muscles. At the same time look for any discomfort the client experiences throughout the ROM. This may be seen as flinching, a change in expression, or verbal cues. Resisted ROM can also be used to assess overall strength of the musculature.

COMMON APPROACHES

OUTLINE

Basic Swedish Massage
   Touch without Movement
   Effleurage
   Pétrissage
   Friction
   Tapotement
   Vibration
   Joint Movements
Structural Bodywork
Myofascial Approach
   Fascia
Trigger-Point Therapy
   Trigger Points
Friction Techniques
Stretching
Putting it all Together

KEY TERMS

ballistic stretching
connective tissue
dynamic stretching
effleurage
friction
Hellerwork
ischemia
joint movements
myofascial massage
myofascial release
pétrissage
Rolfing
static stretching
structural integration
tapotement
thixotropy
touch without movement
trigger point
vibration

OBJECTIVES

1   Define the seven basic massage strokes.
2   Understand the modalities that influence deep tissue massage.

Although deep tissue massage is often listed as a specific modality, it is more like an intention or approach to reach a specific goal. In William Shakespeare's *Romeo and Juliet,* Juliet says, "What's in a name? That which we call a rose by any other name would smell as sweet." A technique is a technique, no matter how we classify it. For example, applying digital compression, be it for structural work, myofascial release, Swedish massage, or sports massage, is still digital compression. What changes is the intention or purpose behind the stroke. You can change the speed, pressure, angle, or drag to get a different result. Deep tissue massage builds on the basic massage techniques to reach a specific layer of tissue and outcome. To better understand deep tissue massage, this chapter reviews some of the history and theories of massage approaches.

BASIC SWEDISH MASSAGE

History tells us that the roots of massage are well grounded in culture and tradition. Written accounts of massage show that it has been around for more than 5,000 years and can be found in every culture around the world. Pehr Henrik Ling (1776-1839) is credited with many developments and systemized routines known as *medical gymnastics* (Figure 3-1). These included active

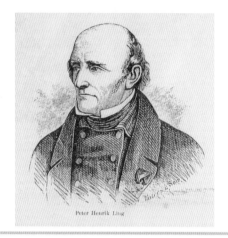

FIGURE 3-1 ■ Pehr Henrik Ling (1776-1839). Father of physical therapy and Swedish massage. (Courtesy Calvert RN: *The history of massage: an illustrated survey from around the world.* Rochester, 2002, Healing Arts Press.)

and passive movements like exercise, stroking, shaking, hacking, and squeezing. Dr. Johann Mezger (1839-1909) coined the French terms *effleurage, pétrissage, friction,* and *tapotement* to describe these movements, and brought them to the scientific community.

Therapists build on these basic techniques to address musculoskeletal complaints. These techniques can be classified into seven categories used in the Western approach: touch without movement, effleurage, pétrissage, friction, tapotement, vibration, and joint movements.

TOUCH WITHOUT MOVEMENT

Touch without movement is often overlooked or not defined as an important technique in the massage industry. This technique is applied to the body without visible movement. For example, therapists commonly hold the client's head and touch the back or feet at the beginning and end of the session for a lasting comfort and calming effect. Another important approach in this category is *direct* or *static pressure.* These are commonly used in deep tissue massage and in craniosacral, myofascial, and trigger-point approaches. Direct pressure has often been classified as "touch without movement" because of the compression it creates. It is effective because it causes the fascial system to melt and unwind, and because it creates **ischemia** at a particular location (Figure 3-2).

EFFLEURAGE

Effleurage is defined as sliding or gliding strokes over the body with a continuous motion. *Gliding, stripping, broadening,* and *stroking* are common terms used to define techniques that fall under this category. Effleurage is one of the most

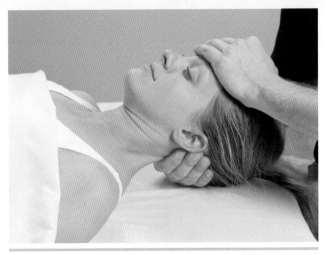

FIGURE 3-2 ■ Touch without movement.

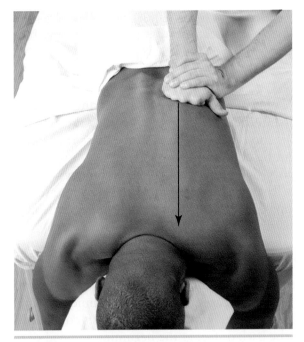

FIGURE 3-3 ■ Effleurage.

versatile and most used techniques by massage therapists. These techniques can be used not only to spread lubricants and as a transitioning stroke, but can also be used to create specific changes within the musculoskeletal system (Figure 3-3).

PÉTRISSAGE

Pétrissage strokes involve lifting, kneading, and squeezing the tissues of the body. Kneading, squeezing, skin rolling, and some compression techniques can be classified under pétrissage. The focus of pétrissage techniques is to press or move the tissues between the hands to aid in breaking up adhesions and loosen the muscle fibers (Figure 3-4).

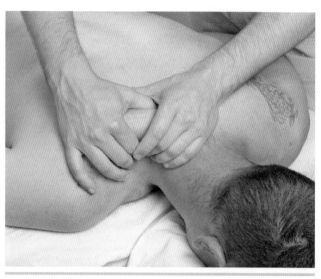

FIGURE 3-4 ▥ Pétrissage.

FRICTION

Friction describes techniques that move one surface over another in a repetitive motion. Friction can take place at many depths within the body. Deep friction addresses the more internal layers of tissue, whereas superficial friction addresses the outer layers. Longitudinal friction is applied with the fiber of the muscle, whereas transverse or cross-fiber friction is applied against the grain of the muscle. Friction can also be applied in a circular or multidirectional pattern. Multidirectional friction is an effective technique when working with scar tissue (Figure 3-5).

TAPOTEMENT

Tapotement consists of quick, repetitive, rhythmic motions used to stimulate tissues. Some tapotement techniques like cupping are often referred to as *percussion* or *percussive techniques.* Percussive techniques include tapping, hacking, beating, cupping, and pincement (Figure 3-6).

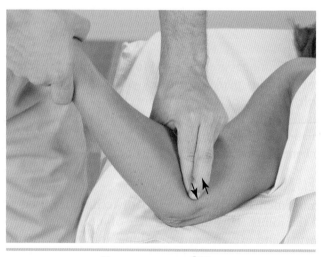

FIGURE 3-5 ▥ Friction.

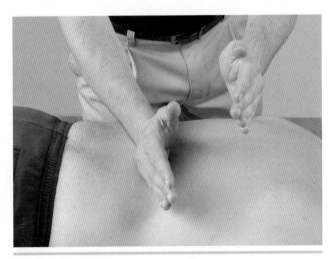

FIGURE 3-6 ▪ Tapotement.

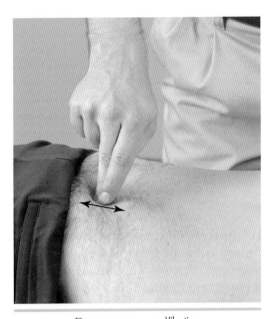

FIGURE 3-7 ▪ Vibration.

VIBRATION

Vibration techniques are similar to friction and tapotement in that they involve rhythmic motions performed quickly. These motions are performed in back-and-forth, circular, or quivering movements and involve shaking and jostling the muscle or quivering over a nerve trunk. Vibration is intended to be used as a stimulating technique that can help "wake up" a muscle or bring an awareness to the client of what that part of the body feels like (Figure 3-7).

JOINT MOVEMENTS

Joint movements involve a variety of techniques used to loosen the tissues around the joints. This includes range-of-motion, active, passive, and resistive movements, and exercise and stretching. Joint movements or range of motion (ROM) exercises as discussed in Chapter 2 can be used for assessment, but the movement can also create several therapeutic responses. Joint movements help

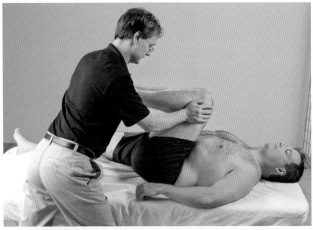

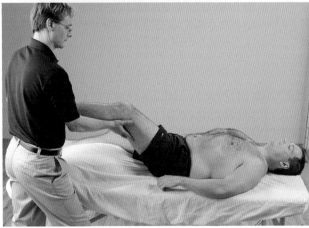

FIGURE 3-8 ■ Joint movement.

activate the proprioceptors of the body. Joint receptors, muscle spindle cells, and Golgi tendon organs are stimulated during movements at the joint. Joint movements also help lubricate the joints and set neurologic pathways to support and strengthen the joints (Figure 3-8).

These techniques can be adjusted, combined, or manipulated to achieve a certain therapeutic response. According to the "Bodywork Glossary" on the Massage Therapy Information website, there are more than 200 different modalities for massage and bodywork. All of these modalities stem from these basic classifications of movement. There are different intentions and approaches to using these techniques; however, the technique itself is the mechanism used to create the outcome.

Deep tissue massage is based on the combination of these seven basic strokes with the intention of reaching the deeper layers of tissues in the body. It blends the theories of multiple modalities to achieve a session that provides deep therapeutic relief.

STRUCTURAL BODYWORK

Structural bodywork stems from the development of osteopathic medicine in the early 1900s. Rolfing, **Hellerwork**, the Trager method, and the Feldenkrais method are a few common modalities that focus on structural and postural alignment.

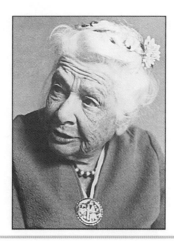

FIGURE 3-9 ■ Ida Pauline Rolf, PhD (May 18, 1896–March 19, 1979). "God didn't come down and tell me; I had to find it out through many years of experience. The work came first; the inspiration came later." (Photo by David Kirk-Campbell).

One of the goals of these modalities is to use the **connective tissues** of the body to aid in the proper alignment of posture and biomechanics. Two major founders and contributors to structural bodywork modalities are Elizabeth Dicke and Ida Rolf (Figure 3-9).

Elizabeth Dicke was a German physiotherapist credited with developing a connective-tissue approach that focused on the superficial connective tissue of the body. This approach was designed to help clients with pathologic conditions of the vascular and visceral systems. The theory is that working the superficial fascia loosens and removes adhesions surrounding the muscles, blood and lymph vessels, and the nerves. This allows the fluids to flow freely throughout the body, helps increase range of motion and flexibility, and releases taut tissues.

Ida Rolf's involvement with structural bodywork began when she worked with osteopaths in the 1930s. What started as **structural integration** later became known as **Rolfing** because her students talked about "getting Rolfed" when she worked on them. Rolfing's focus is on correcting the ill effects of constant poor posture and gravitational effects on the body. It focuses on the deeper fascia of the body to realign the body into a position that can withstand the gravitational pressure put on the joints. Traditionally this form of bodywork requires 10 specific sessions.

These two leaders in the structural bodywork approach paved the way for many others to develop similar approaches with a focus on the fascial and connective tissues of the body to aid in proper structural and postural alignment. Contributors to furthering the development of structural integration approach include Joseph Heller, Judith Aston, and Thomas Myers.

MYOFASCIAL APPROACH

Myofascial massage is a classification of modalities that includes techniques that focus on the fascial connection throughout the body. This category includes **myofascial release**, unwinding, and other fascial approaches that focus

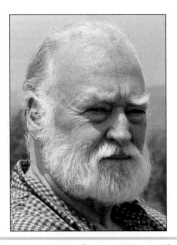

FIGURE 3-10 ■ John F. Barnes, PT, LMT, NCTMB (February 3, 1939–). "The master therapist is real, calm, nonjudgmental, intelligent, sensitive, strong yet flexible, supportive, compassionate, empathic, and joyful." (Courtesy John F. Barnes. In Salvo SG: *Massage therapy: principles and practice,* ed 4, St Louis, 2012, Saunders.)

on releasing restrictions found in the different layers of the fascial matrix. This approach has developed over time along with the developments of Bindegewebs and Rolfing. Robert Ward is credited with coining the term *myofascial release* in the 1960s, but John Barnes made the technique more popular and easily accessible to the massage therapist in the 1980s (Figure 3-10). Many methods continue to develop based on these approaches to myofascial massage and are becoming more commonplace in therapists' skills.

FASCIA

To better understand the effects of myofascial modalities and their role in deep tissue massage, it is important to understand fascia and its role in the body. Fascia is a three-dimensional matrix of loose connective tissue that surrounds bone, muscle, visceral organs, and skin, providing shape, support, and connections throughout the body. Composed of three substances, this matrix connects the big toe to the top of the skull. Collagen provides fascia with strong and flexible protein fibers, which is the most common fiber in connective tissues. Elastin fibers allow fascia to return to its original length and aid fascia elasticity. Ground substance is a gel that fills the spaces among the fibers to help hydrate and keep the fascia pliable.

Fascia displays an interesting property called *thixotropy.* **Thixotropy** is the ability to change from a solid to a more liquid state. Three main components are needed to help fascia move to a more liquid and pliable state: hydration, heat, and movement. Within the fascial matrix of elastin and collagen fibers is a gel-like fluid known as *ground substance.* This gel, when cold relative to the temperature of the body, becomes more viscous. *Viscosity* is a resistance to flow. Something with a higher viscosity becomes thicker when cold, making it harder to move. In the case of fascial and joint mobility, the warmer the tissue, the more pliable it becomes.

TRIGGER-POINT THERAPY

Trigger-point therapy has become a common therapeutic approach. The use of trigger-point therapy to address common muscular complaints can be traced back to Stanley Lief, but became popular in the United States with the advancements of Dr. Janet Travell. Travell popularized the terms *trigger points* and *referral patterns* and published her findings in "The Myofascial Genesis of Pain" in 1952. Dr. Travell used her trigger-point approach to help President John F. Kennedy's pain and later worked with President Lyndon Johnson, which brought national attention to trigger-point therapy (Figure 3-11). The work of Bonnie Prudden has brought the practice of locating and relieving trigger points to the general public.

Trigger-point therapy addresses specific areas of hyperirritability located within the muscles and connective tissue. This approach involves locating these trigger points and deactivating them.

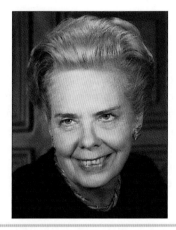

FIGURE 3-11 ▪ Janet Travell, MD (December 17, 1901–August 1, 1997). "It is obvious that our potential for optimal health depends not alone on the pathology of disease, but on the fiber of our personalities." (From Salvo SG: *Massage therapy: principles and practice,* ed 4, St Louis, 2012, Saunders.)

TRIGGER POINTS

Trigger points can manifest in the connective tissues and are caused by a variety of sources. Trauma and postural habits can cause muscles to contract to protect and keep the body in balance. Repetitive movements and ergonomics add stress to muscles, potentially overloading them. Disease and disorders can also indirectly affect the connective tissue, resulting in trigger points.

Active trigger points are areas of hypersensitivity and, when compressed, refer pain and discomfort. These points are consistently tender or sore even at rest and often twitch when pressed. Active trigger points show symptoms in an area that can be distant from the site of irritability. These symptoms are often experienced as numbness, tingling, aching, or burning.

Latent trigger points are areas of hyperirritability that do not elicit referral pain or can be felt only in the area of the trigger point. Most clients are unaware of these areas of hyperirritability as they are sore only when touched. These points are commonly recognized by the client with the comment, "I didn't know I was sore there." Latent trigger points may become active with daily activity, postural disorders, or overuse of the muscle. These points generally do not refer pain until they become active; however, they do create dysfunctions such as muscle weakness and loss of range of motion.

There are several approaches to treating trigger points. Some of the more effective techniques are ischemic compression, positional release, and muscle energy techniques.

FRICTION TECHNIQUES

As discussed earlier in this chapter, friction is the rubbing of two surfaces together. This technique can be performed at various levels of depth. Superficial friction helps to increase circulation and generates heat. These are two important effects in the process of healing and working with body alignment. Techniques like superficial friction, rolling, and wringing are effective in addressing the superficial fascia of the body.

Popularized by James Cyriax, deep transverse friction took the massage profession to new levels. This approach, also known as *cross-fiber friction*, is applied perpendicular to the fibers of the tissue. For this, it is important that the therapist have a strong understanding of the muscle and fiber direction. Commonly applied to the muscle belly, this technique helps to break adhesions by broadening the tissue and realigning the fibers. It is also effective with the tendons and ligaments of the body (Figure 3-12).

Circular friction can be applied to specific areas and is usually used around bony landmarks and joints. This approach uses small circular movements to increase the flow of fluids, create heat, and help to realign fibers.

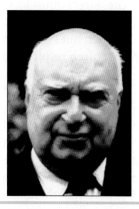

FIGURE 3-12 ■ James Henry Cyriax, MD, MRCP (1904–June 17, 1985). Physician, father of orthopedic medicine. "He could often be seen walking backwards along Lambeth Palace Road round to the bus stop on Westminster Bridge so as to keep an eye on the oncoming buses." (From Salvo SG: *Massage therapy: principles and practice,* ed 4, St Louis, 2012, Saunders.)

Longitudinal friction is a term commonly used for "with grain" friction. This technique applies friction in the same direction as the fibers of the tissues being worked. This approach is most often applied to tissues in the extremities where cross-fiber or circular friction is not possible, like the hands or feet.

Multidirectional friction is becoming more common in the field of fascial work. As discussed earlier, fascial research is growing and new developments are surfacing around effective techniques for fascial massage. One of these developments is based on the understanding that the collagen fibers of fascia exist in a multidirectional pattern. For this reason, working with deep friction in a multidirectional approach has shown better results than transverse friction alone.

STRETCHING

Stretching is crucial to the overall health of the body. Stretching helps increase flexibility and remove adhesions, and allows the body to move more fluidly. The process of stretching involves the elongation of the muscle through a full range of motion. It is important to understand the mechanics and functions of the muscle that is being stretched and the joint that it acts on. If performed aggressively or if the wrong method is used, stretching can cause potential damage to the client's tissues.

Static stretching is a safe and effective stretch. Most people are familiar with these stretches and often perform them at home. Bob Anderson popularized this approach to stretching in his book, *Stretching*. Static stretching is a slow and progressive elongation of the target muscle by holding the stretch for 15-30 seconds. At this point the person can progress further into the stretch and hold again.

Ballistic stretching, although popular, can be detrimental to the body. This type of stretching is often referred to as a type of **dynamic stretching** and was practiced by athletes for years. Ballistic stretching involves rapid bouncing motions to force the target muscle to elongate. These rapid bouncing motions can cause the muscles to contract as a protective reflex and may result in microtrauma to the tissues. These microtears in the tissues, along with the muscular contractions, often result in the target muscle becoming taut and restricted.

Passive stretching is one of the most controlled forms of stretching and is used by many therapists and rehabilitation specialists. This form of stretching usually involves a therapist controlling the stretch through a specific motion. The client relaxes to the point of the elongation and the therapist can then progress the movement throughout its range of motion.

Proprioceptive neuromuscular facilitation (PNF) is a common passive technique practiced by massage therapists and athletic trainers. PNF uses the neuromuscular stretch reflex to increase range of motion and to reeducate the body. Common techniques used in PNF are the contract-relax and antagonist-contraction techniques, and a combination of both known as the contract-relax-antagonist contraction technique.

The contract-relax technique uses the postisometric relaxation technique, in which the agonist muscle is contracted for a short duration. Immediately following this contraction, there is a period during which all neural impulses are inhibited to that muscle, allowing it to relax. This relaxation period is ideal for progressing further into the stretch. The antagonist contraction is based on the reciprocal inhibition technique, which means that while the antagonist muscle is contracting, the agonist muscle must be relaxed because of the nervous inhibition. When combined, these neurologic laws allow the therapist to move into a stretch, have the client contract against a resistance, and then actively move into a position of a deeper stretch.

PUTTING IT ALL TOGETHER

As with all forms of bodywork, there is a progression of working through layers to access the deeper underlying tissues. When working with connective tissues, it is important to remember that the keys to creating a change in the tissues and alignment of fibers lie not only in the techniques but also in the approach.

Every successful session follows a sequence. Therapists should start with general techniques, moving to specific areas and finishing with general techniques often referred to as *transitional techniques*. This pattern can be applied to other sequencing as well. Sessions start with general strokes moving in a proximal direction, then specific techniques working distally. General techniques are best applied superficially, whereas specific techniques are applied in a smaller and deeper approach. When working with an area of hypersensitivity, it is often best to work around the area first and progress to the core rather than starting directly on the point of irritation (Table 3-1).

Before working the deeper tissues of the body, it is crucial to make sure the superficial layers are warmed up and that their issues have been addressed. Keep in mind that the deeper your strokes go, the slower the technique should become. Because of the pressure involved, tissues, structures, and visceral organs can easily be injured. These approaches to deep tissue need to be performed with focus and intention. Pressure creates friction and this friction creates heat. As the tissue becomes warmer, the ground substance becomes less viscous, which is beneficial when working to realign muscle fibers and enhancing pliability.

Table 3-1 **PROGRESSION OF APPROACH**

	STARTING	DETAIL WORK	TRANSITIONING TO NEXT AREA
Strokes	General	Specific	General
Direction	Proximal	Distal	Proximal
Pressure	Superficial	Deep	Superficial
Hypersensitive Areas	Edges	Core	Edges

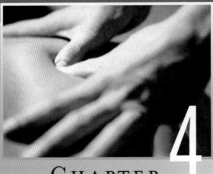

CHAPTER 4

TOOLS AND TECHNIQUES

OBJECTIVES

1   Explain and demonstrate the principles of deep tissue massage.
2   Apply deep tissue techniques.
3   Explain the parts of the body commonly used for deep tissue massage.
4   Demonstrate how to use the body to apply appropriate techniques.

KEY TERMS

body mechanics
depth
functional anatomy
intention
interphalangeal (IP) joint
kinesiology
layer
metacarpophalangeal (MCP) joint
muscle belly
neutral position
nonverbal communication
physiology
principles of deep tissue massage
speed
superficial
verbal communication
withdraw

Deep tissue massage focuses on the deeper tissues of the body. It does not mean that the therapist needs to apply more pressure to access these tissues. Therapists who consistently use stronger pressure to perform deep tissue massage are putting themselves and their clients at risk for injury. Repetitive and strong forces on the therapist's joints can lead to long-term trauma and shorten the career of the therapist. The strong pressure being applied to the client can result in bruising, pain, and discomfort for the client and may lead to long-term muscle damage. In this chapter we explore ways to use different parts of the body to provide the "strong pressure" feeling without having to exert more energy. Using the fists, elbows, forearms, or knuckles can meet the needs and goals of the session while protecting the therapist from stress and injuries.

Deep tissue massage is experienced differently by everybody. Hypersensitivity and pain thresholds vary from person to person. One client may prefer that you use your elbow along the medial border of the scapula, whereas another client may feel the palm is strong enough. Smooth application of **depth** and pressure depends on the therapist's abilities to recognize verbal and nonverbal communication.

In **verbal communication** the client provides verbal feedback such as "It is tender there" or "More pressure." Some clients prefer not to talk during a session, making verbal communication challenging. Prompting your client with questions like "Is that tender?" "How is my pressure?" or "Does that provide relief?" becomes important for the therapist.

Nonverbal communication is observed through body language, posture, and gestures. Although the client may be requesting more pressure, the therapist may feel tension in the muscle or the body might twitch. The ability to recognize nonverbal communication is important in deep tissue massage. The therapist needs to recognize changes in facial expression, slight adjustments on the table, or tightening of the muscle, as these are all signs of discomfort. Changes in breath and changes in texture of the muscle help guide the therapist on the effectiveness of the technique.

PRINCIPLES OF DEEP TISSUE MASSAGE

It is better to work smarter rather than harder. Understanding the approach to accessing the deeper layers of tissue and how to appropriately use the body provides a longer and safer career for the therapist. Following are some key **principles of deep tissue massage** to remember when working with the deeper layers of tissues, which will help to facilitate this work.

Be cautious of the use of lubricants when going deep. Lubricants are used to prevent friction on the skin during massage. Too much lubrication can prevent the therapist from hooking or grabbing the tissue, forcing the therapist to work harder. Hooking into the skin for stretching is important and too much oil or cream may interfere with a good stretch. Using excessive amounts of a lubricant may also cause the therapist to slide off the muscle during the technique. This may cause the muscle to snap back into place, which causes pain to the client because of the sudden shift in location of the pressure.

Deep tissue work should be slow. The deeper the stroke, the slower it should become. This allows the therapist to focus on what he or she is doing, the position he or she is working, and the goal of the technique. Pain commonly associated with deeper work is not caused by the pressure being used, but the **speed** of the stroke. Broad, deep, and fast work stimulates the sympathetic rather than the parasympathetic nervous system. Stimulation of the parasympathetic nervous system is necessary for muscle relaxation. A slower stroke aids in better identification of changes in the muscle texture and locating trigger points.

Focus on the layer you are working and work that layer. The body has multiple **layers** of muscles and each muscle has its specific role. **Superficial** muscles engage to create movements, whereas the deeper muscles focus on stability and support. The body is aware of where the therapist is working and sudden shifts from layer to layer can confuse the body. If you work each layer completely and move to the next, you will be able to feel the change in the muscle tissue when it has relaxed. This is where a plan becomes important. Working the superficial gluteus muscles, then moving to the piriformis, then back to the gluteals, then to the quadratus femoris, and then back the gluteals can be confusing and taxing to the nervous system. If there is no release from the superficial muscles, going deeper can lead to discomfort to the client and may result in increased muscular tension and possible bruising. It is best to work the superficial layer completely and then progress to the deeper layers.

When completing an area of deep massage, do not just withdraw the stroke. When pulling out of the layers of tissues, the speed must be slow. Sudden movements when working and exiting an area can trigger a protective mechanism and cause muscles to contract. This contraction, similar to the twitch response, can create the tension you just released. Smooth out the area before moving on to the next. Effleurage stroke helps normalize circulation in the area just worked and calms the nervous system.

Use the right tool for the right technique. Many therapists depend on physical strength to reach the deeper structures of the body. The therapist should use his or her body position, proper **body mechanics**, and tools to achieve this goal without adding to the stress on his or her own body (Box 4-1).

Box 4-1　**PRINCIPLES OF DEEP TISSUE MASSAGE**

1. Limit use of lubricants.
2. The deeper the work, the slower the technique.
3. Work the layers.
4. Withdraw cautiously.
5. Choose the right tool for the technique.

TOOLS FOR DEEP TISSUE MASSAGE

The most important tools therapists have are their minds and bodies. Knowledge and understanding of anatomy, physiology, and kinesiology are important tools for deep tissue massage. **Intention** is the mental determination of a specific action or result. Having a clear intention directly influences the approach and outcomes of the session.

It is important to determine why deep tissue massage is being used during a session. Is the therapist applying deep tissue massage to access a deeper layer of musculature or is it being applied for the pressure that the client is requesting? Clients can receive a massage session that is more intense in pressure without going into the deep musculature of the body. Strong knowledge in **functional**

anatomy and **physiology** helps direct the therapist in the assessment and evaluation of the client's current position or situation. Applying the knowledge of anatomy and **kinesiology** assists in establishing the appropriate approach and techniques necessary to reach the outcomes of the session. The client intake; health assessment; postural and gait analysis; and subjective, objective, assessment, and plan notes help clarify how the body is affected by activities of daily living and how it is reacting to the massage techniques being used.

Use of the body is crucial for safe and effective applications of deep tissue massage. Building on the skills learned in massage training regarding body mechanics, there is little difference between classical massage body positioning and deep tissue positioning. One of the first adjustments therapists commonly make is setting up the table. To apply proper leverage and to adjust body positioning, it is common for deep tissue therapists to set the table height a notch or two lower than normal. This may allow the therapist to use more leverage and body weight to apply pressure. A lower table also allows easier access for the therapist to kneel or get on the table if needed. Be aware of where your weight is and how you use your body weight to achieve the pressure necessary. Changing your stance by taking a longer or shorter stance with a lower table may be necessary.

Some deep tissue practitioners prefer to raise the table a notch. This higher table allows the therapist to use the forearms and elbows more efficiently and with less stress on the back. Either way, the table height needs to be adjusted to a height that is both comfortable for the therapist and appropriate for the preferred technique.

ARMS AND ELBOWS

The forearm is a great tool to use when administering compression or gliding strokes over a larger area. The forearm provides two surface areas to use based on the technique and desired results. Using the ulnar surface of the forearm provides a harder surface when compressing or broadening strokes are used in areas of dense musculature. It also provides a softer surface when using the muscular side of the forearm, which is beneficial in areas of thinner muscles (Figure 4-1).

Muscle compression with the forearm allows for the pressure to be administered over a large, broad surface. The forearm also provides a tool that can easily be adjusted based on the client's needs. The **muscle belly** of the flexors of the wrist and digits are in the forearm. During forearm compression some therapists make a fist and squeeze to adjust the firmness in the forearm. Although this clenching and unclenching of the hand affects the amount of pressure felt by the client, it can be dangerous to the therapist. Tightening the fist and wrist expends more energy, fatigues the forearm, and potentially leads to long-term injuries. It is better to supinate or pronate the forearm to create the same feeling. As the therapist supinates the forearm, he or she is shifting more toward the ulnar surface of the forearm, providing a harder surface; the more pronated the forearm, the more he or she are using the muscular flexor muscles, creating a softer surface.

It is important for therapists to become comfortable with using the forearm and the diversity it offers. Using the forearm takes stress off the wrist and finger and allows the therapist to offer more pressure with less effort. It can be used for

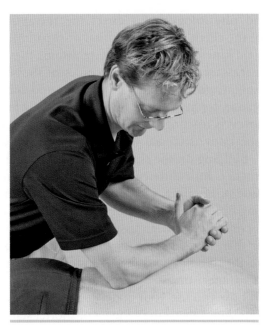

FIGURE 4-1 ■ Forearm.

gliding strokes, specifically for stripping strokes for larger areas. The forearm can also be used as a compressive tool when compressing a larger area is necessary.

The elbow is another valuable tool for applying compressive forces to the body. The elbow allows the therapist to apply compression to a specific, defined area of the body. The elbow is the best tool to alleviate the stress applied to the thumb during many compressive techniques, especially in areas where there is large muscle density. Be cautious that the smaller surface area of the elbow in relation to the forearm creates a different sensation of pressure. The elbow is a harder surface than the forearm, which creates the sensation of increased pressure to the client. When using the elbow, less pressure is often needed to get the same result (Figure 4-2).

As the therapist uses the elbows more, it is important to adapt the body mechanics to a new position. Application of the elbows brings the therapist closer to the client's body and requires the therapist to lean more into the client. Longer stances and good posture are keys to avoid undue stress on the therapist's lumbar spine. The ulnar nerve is superficial in this area of the arm. Improper use of the elbow may compress this nerve, causing numbness or tingling in the therapist's arm. If the therapist is experiencing these sensations, he or she should try repositioning the elbow using a different surface or discontinue using this technique completely.

HANDS

The most common tool the therapist uses is the hands. Most therapists use their palms, fingers, and thumbs throughout the massage session. Prolonged use can lead to cumulative damage and may shorten a therapist's career. Using different surfaces of the hands during deep tissue massage becomes more important because of the increased stress on the joints.

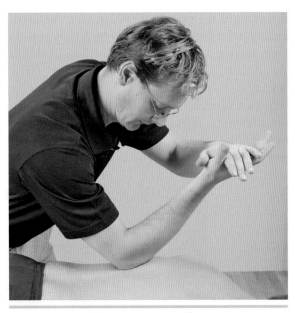

FIGURE 4-2 ▨ Elbow.

The fist offers the therapist a surface to use while keeping the wrist in a **neutral position**. Fists can be used to apply compressive strokes or gliding strokes. It offers a surface area that is larger than the elbow, yet not as broad as the forearm. This is advantageous when stripping muscles like the hamstrings and erector group. The fist allows the therapist to apply firm pressure without getting too close to the client, unlike the elbow and forearms (Figure 4-3).

Fists can be applied in two positions: open or closed. With an open fist, the therapist flexes only at the **metacarpophalangeal (MCP) joints**. This position allows the therapist to keep the flexor muscles relaxed and allows the knuckles

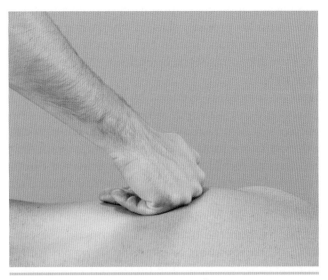

FIGURE 4-3 ▨ Fist.

and dorsal surface of the proximal phalanges to be used. With a closed fist, the therapist makes a fist by flexing both the MCP and the **interphalangeal (IP) joints**. When making a closed fist, the tension in the forearm increases, which can lead to quicker fatigue. The closed fist allows for more comfort using the knuckle surface.

Use of fists and knuckles is beneficial for stripping strokes, compression, and compressive stretching. It is important to keep the wrist in a neutral position; flexion or extension at the wrist during these movements adds stress to the wrist joint and may cause trauma and discomfort (Figure 4-4).

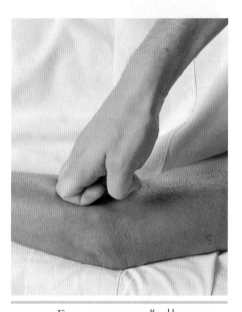

FIGURE 4-4 ■ Knuckle.

Knuckles are another tool that assist in alleviating the stress and fatigue in the fingers and hands. Therapists should try to use their knuckles rather than their thumb when applying compression or deep glides. It is important to make sure all the joints are properly stacked when using the knuckles. The wrist must be in a neutral position, not in flexion-extension and adduction-abduction. Failure to have the joints stacked results in increased pressure at the MCP and at the wrist joints.

Fingers are commonly overused by massage therapists. Fingers are beneficial for palpation and assessment of structures and tissues. The fingertips provide a small surface area, which allows for specific detailed work. Fingers and fingertips are the therapist's most diverse tool. Compression, friction, squeezing, and tapotement are all techniques that can be delivered through the fingers. Their diversity explains why therapists tend to overuse them (Figure 4-5).

When using the fingers during deep tissue work, it is important to add support to protect the joints and prevent trauma and fatigue. This can be achieved by using fingers from the other hand to support the position or by adding a finger in an overlay position. Strength in the fingers is built over time, but it is important to properly support the fingers or to use a different position like the closed fist to take advantage of the knuckle surface to prevent fatigue and injury.

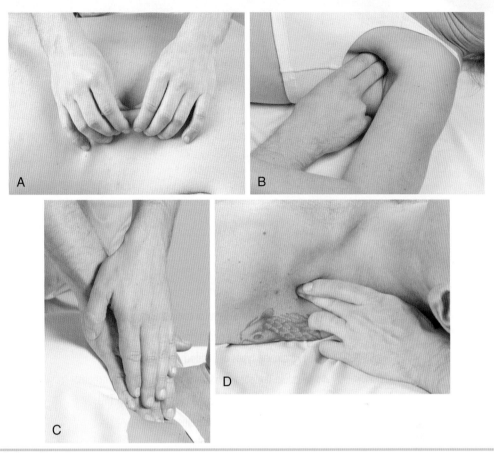

FIGURE 4-5 ■ Fingers. **A**, Muscle squeezing. **B**, Digital compression. **C**, Digital compression with support. **D**, Finger with overlay position.

MASSAGE TOOLS

Throughout history, cultures have used tools to aid in the treatment of muscular soreness. In time, massage tools have been redesigned to match technologies, knowledge, and materials available. Whether the tools are made from wood, stone, or plastic, they have been used to help the therapist prevent injury and to aid in the massage session. Massage tools also function as a way for both the therapist and the client to administer self-help treatments between sessions.

Stone massage tools have the ability to be heated or cooled, hard tools can be used as an alternative to fingers or knuckles, and sticks and flexible tools can be used for tapotement. There are a wide variety of electronic tools that can be used as vibratory devices. Although there are thousands of devices available to the therapist, caution should be used with these tools.

When using an external tool to aid in massage, there is a disconnection between the therapist and client. The therapist is working through an object that may diffuse the sensations of changes in the client's body. When working with the deeper layers of tissues or in areas of hypersensitivity, attention to these subtle changes is important and the use of tools may interfere with this awareness.

CHAPTER 5

HEAD AND NECK

KEY TERMS

atlas (C1)
axis (C2)
body position
brachial plexus
carotid artery
central nervous system
cervical plexus
cervical vertebrae
congenital torticollis
exertional and tension headache
headaches (HAs)
jugular vein
migraine
organic headache
spasmodic torticollis (ST)
temporomandibular joint (TMJ)
thoracic outlet syndrome (TOS)
toxic headache
whiplash

OBJECTIVES

1   Understand the structural components of the cervical region.
2   Be knowledgeable about the effects position has on the head and neck.
3   Explain the types of headaches.
4   Explain temporomandibular joint (TMJ) dysfunctions.
5   Understand the effects the muscles have on TMJ.
6   Explain the types of torticollis.
7   Explain the causes of whiplash.
8   Define *thoracic outlet syndrome.*

The area of the head and neck is one of the most complex and overworked regions in the body. At some point in their lives most people will complain about a pain in their neck. Because of its structure and function, it is easy to understand why neck pain is so prevalent. Imagine a semisolid base holding a rod arced at 30-40 degrees, which supports a 10-pound bowling ball. This is the structure of the neck. The base of the neck is the torso, which consists of the thoracic vertebrae, rib cage, and sternum. The arced rod consists of the seven cervical vertebrae and their intervertebral discs. The bowling ball represents the head, which weighs an average of 8-10 pounds (Figure 5-1).

The cervical area has sacrificed structure to provide mobility, including extension, flexion, lateral flexion, rotations, and many combinations of these movements. This area is rich in nerves, ligaments, and musculature. The complex musculature of the neck is necessary for stabilization of the head, to maintain its balance, and to control these movements (Figure 5-2).

Anterior atlanto-occipital membrane
Anterior arch of atlas (C1)
Tectorial membrane
Cruciate ligament of dens
Occiput
Axis (C2)
Posterior atlanto-occipital ligament
Posterior tuberale of atlas (C1)
Posterior longitudinal ligament
Anterior longitudinal ligament
Supraspinous ligament
Facet joint capsules
Nuchal ligament
Body of C4
Ligamenta flava
Intervertebral discs
C7 spinous process
Interspinous ligament

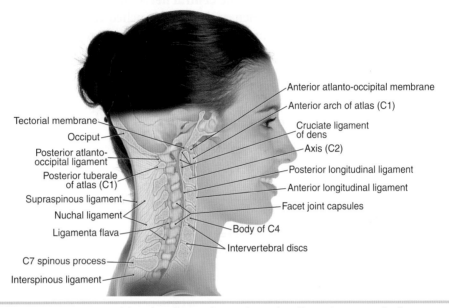

FIGURE 5-1 ■ Structure of the neck. (From Muscolino JE: *The muscle and bone palpation manual with trigger points, referral patterns, and stretching*, St Louis, 2009, Mosby.)

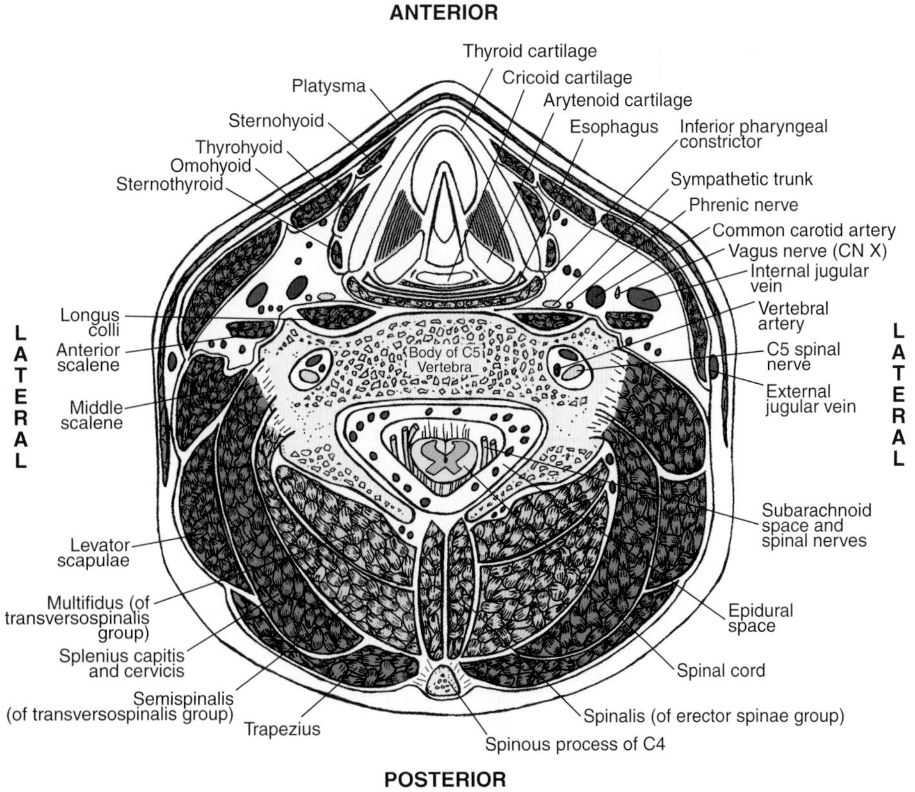

ANTERIOR
Thyroid cartilage
Platysma
Cricoid cartilage
Arytenoid cartilage
Sternohyoid
Esophagus
Inferior pharyngeal constrictor
Thyrohyoid
Omohyoid
Sternothyroid
Sympathetic trunk
Phrenic nerve
Common carotid artery
Vagus nerve (CN X)
Internal jugular vein
Longus colli
Vertebral artery
LATERAL
Anterior scalene
Body of C5 Vertebra
C5 spinal nerve
LATERAL
External jugular vein
Middle scalene
Subarachnoid space and spinal nerves
Levator scapulae
Multifidus (of transversospinalis group)
Epidural space
Splenius capitis and cervicis
Spinal cord
Semispinalis (of transversospinalis group)
Spinalis (of erector spinae group)
Trapezius
Spinous process of C4
POSTERIOR

FIGURE 5-2 ■ Cross-section of the neck. (From Muscolino JE: *The muscular system manual: the skeletal muscles of the human body*, ed 3, St Louis, 2010, Mosby.)

The cervical spine is a complex area that also requires extreme caution because of its vascularization and nerves. The obvious concern while working with any region of the spine is the **central nervous system**. The spinal cord runs through the vertebral foramen and can be pinched or damaged with forceful movements. Although damage to the spinal cord is rare with therapeutic massage, the peripheral nerves, such as the **cervical plexus** (C1-C4) and **brachial plexus** (C5-C8) as they exit the spine, are susceptible to damage in massage therapy. Innervations from the cervical plexus feed the face and neck with the stimulus needed for movement and function. The brachial plexus feeds the arms and hands with their needed stimuli (Figure 5-3).

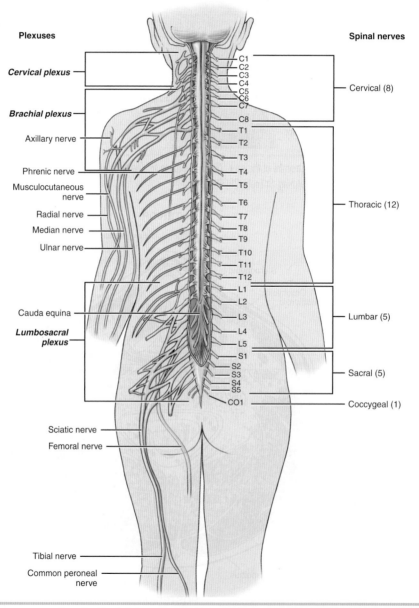

FIGURE 5-3 ■ Cervical and brachial plexus. (From Herlihy B: *The human body in health and illness,* ed 4, St Louis, 2011, Saunders.)

The vascular design in the cervical region raises additional concerns. **Cervical vertebrae** 1 through 6 contain a transverse foramen, which provides a protected pathway to the brain for the vertebral artery and vein. Because of the motion, especially rotation of the neck, this is a high-risk area. Rotating the neck to access tissues or applying a stretch can apply pressure to these vessels, which can result in fainting, nausea, and vertigo. This potential to pinch or compress the vertebral artery happens at approximately 45-50 degrees of rotation. On the anterior aspect of the neck the **carotid artery** and **jugular vein** hide under the sternocleidomastoid (SCM). The carotid pulse is palpated here as these vessels are superficial in the body. If at any time you are working on the anterior aspects of the neck and feel a pulse, you should change the positioning of your hands (Figure 5-4).

The therapist can place the client in many different **body positions** to address the cervical region. Depending on the muscle being worked, the client can be in a prone, supine, side-lying, or seated position. Each position offers several benefits and disadvantages. The supine position allows the most versatility for assessment of range of motion (ROM) and stretching, also allowing easy access to the anterior neck muscles. From this position the therapist can also access some of the posterior neck muscles. One of the advantages of accessing the posterior neck muscles from this position is that the weight of the head and neck are used as a resistant force, alleviating the need for the therapist to generate the pressure. In the prone position, the face cradle can be a concern. Many face cradles have a cross-bar that can hit the chin or throat when

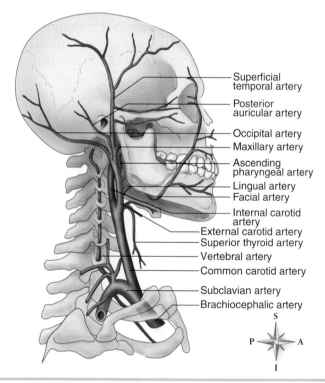

Superficial temporal artery

Posterior auricular artery

Occipital artery
Maxillary artery

Ascending pharyngeal artery
Lingual artery
Facial artery

Internal carotid artery
External carotid artery
Superior thyroid artery
Vertebral artery
Common carotid artery

Subclavian artery
Brachiocephalic artery

FIGURE 5-4 ■ Vessels of the neck. (From Patton KT, Thibodeau GA: *Anatomy & physiology*, ed 8, St Louis, 2013, Mosby.)

downward pressure is applied to the upper back, neck, or head. This pressure on the head can also add pressure to the sinuses and facial bones, which may cause some discomfort. The side-lying position tends to be an underused position. In this position, there is a wide access to anterior, posterior, and lateral musculature of the neck. Side-lying also allows for diversity of joint movements and positioning. Proper support with pillows and bolsters is key to comfort and success in the side-lying position.

MIGRAINES AND HEADACHES

Headaches (HAs) are interesting disorders that affect approximately 90% of the U.S. population every year. *Headaches* are defined as pain in the head originating from a variety of sources. Headaches can originate from the environment (**toxic HA**), stress and tension, vascular engorgement, disease (**organic HA**), and even exercise and strenuous work (**exertional or tension HA**). Research has shown that there are some similarities among the causes of different types of headaches. Many headaches are due to changes in serotonin levels, changes in hormones, and arterial dilation. These changes in the body can be caused by a variety of different stimuli like foods, allergies, muscular tension, body alignment, and hormonal or chemical changes.

In most cases massage is an excellent aid to alleviate headaches. However, it depends on the root cause of the headache. Some headaches, such as organic headaches, can be due to an underlying condition that requires caution before proceeding. If the headache is due to an infection or some form of tumor or other growth, massage is not recommended. If the headache is due to tension or exertion, massage is appropriate. Taking a solid client history and possessing strong palpatory skills aids in differentiation between types of headaches.

TENSION HEADACHES

Tension headaches originate from a mechanical stress or exertion. This could be tightening of the musculature caused by body alignment, poor ergonomics, or stress, among many other things. In most cases, the musculature is overworking to maintain proper alignment of the skull. Although many therapists begin working the trapezius muscles, the root of the muscular tension is typically in the suboccipital muscles. This group of intricate muscles plays an important role in maintaining the balance of the head. They help to stabilize the **atlas (C1)**, **axis (C2)**, and the base of the occiput. As tension builds in the superficial muscles of the body, the suboccipital muscles contract to maintain proper head alignment. Because of the tension on the suboccipital muscles, intervertebral compression may occur in this area, resulting in headaches (Figure 5-5).

Other muscles that play a role in tension headaches are the trapezius, levator scapulae, scalenes, splenius, SCM, and some muscles of the jaw. Each muscle has a pain referral pattern that can help identify the muscles affected. A clear and detailed discussion during the client-intake process helps identify these muscles (Table 5-1).

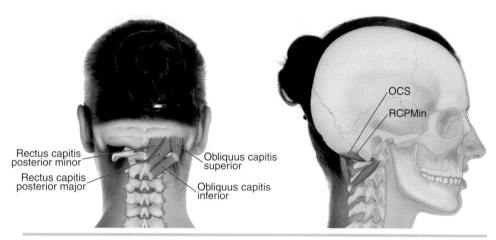

FIGURE 5-5 ■ Suboccipitals. (Muscolino JE: *The muscle and bone palpation manual with trigger points, referral patterns, and stretching*, St Louis, 2009, Mosby.)

Table 5-1 REFERRAL PATTERNS

MUSCLE	REFERRAL PATTERN
Frontalis	Local discomfort occurs above the eye.
Levator scapulae	Refers pain to the base of the neck, top of the shoulder, and vertebral border of the scapula.
Occipitalis	Local discomfort occurs at the back of the head.
Scalene group	Commonly refers pain to the top of the shoulder and down the lateral arm into the first three digits.
Splenius capitis	Refers pain to the top of the head.
Splenius cervicis	Refers pain to the back of the neck and temporal area.
Sternocleidomastoid	Sternal head refers pain to cheek, temporal area, and behind the ear.
	Clavicular head refers pain behind the ear and above the eyes.
Suboccipitals	Refers discomfort in a headband-like area around the eye and above the ears.
Trapezius	Upper fibers refer discomfort to the eye, ear, and lateral neck.

MIGRAINES

Clients often say that there is no experience that comes close to the pain and discomfort of a true migraine. **Migraines** are vascular-based headaches affecting the vessels surrounding the brain. People often experience nausea and vomiting, chills and sweating, extreme fatigue, and visual disturbances. These are often debilitating, causing the person to miss work and stay in bed. Some people experience extreme sensitivity to light and sound. Migraines are often triggered by sensitivity to foods, alcohol, and other drugs, stress, weather changes, sleeping patterns, and posture. They affect women more than men because of hormonal influences (Box 5-1).

Box 5-1 **CONTRAINDICATIONS FOR HEADACHES AND MIGRAINES**

Vascular diseases
Dietary induced migraine
Heart conditions
Advanced diabetes
History of strokes
Vascular migraine
Edema
Cervical herniations
Acute trauma
Peripheral vascular disease

WORKING WITH HEADACHES

Whether the headache is tension related or due to a migraine, caution should be taken before the session. If the client is experiencing a headache, the session should be short, and deep or aggressive techniques should be avoided. Heat should also be avoided, especially if it is a vascular-based headache. Client positioning is also important as the prone position may increase the feeling of pressure in the cranium. Supine positioning may be uncomfortable, depending on the lighting in the room. Clients experiencing light sensitivity may use an eye pillow. A side-lying position is frequently the most comfortable. Remember to support the head and body to the client's level of comfort.

For clients who experience frequent headaches, be sure to take a thorough intake interview, asking about locations of pain during the attack, postural and sleeping habits, food sensitivities, and daily activities. This information helps assess the musculature and postural changes needed to lessen the frequency of headaches.

The focus of the session should be on reducing the trigger points, tight muscles, skeletal imbalances, and increasing ROM of the neck. Work through the layers; start with warming the tissues and the superficial fascia of the area. Address any trigger points or hypertonic tissues found in the upper trapezius muscles. Address the restrictions found in the levator scapulae and SCM using compressive, stripping, and lengthening techniques. As you progress deeper to the splenius and suboccipital muscles, myofascial stretching and compression are effective approaches. Finish the region with joint movements and stretching to help with the neuromuscular reeducation (Sequence 5-1).

TEMPOROMANDIBULAR JOINT DISORDER

Temporomandibular joint (TMJ) disorder is a general term used to describe abnormal functioning of the joint between the temporal bone and the mandible or the jaw. Physicians use this term to classify the symptoms, muscular or skeletal dysfunctions, and common signs associated with the joint at the temporal bone and mandible. Many problems can arise around this joint as it has some unique features. The TMJ is not a true hinge joint. This joint can move up and

Text continued on p. 57

SEQUENCE 5-1

WARM UP OF SUPERFICIAL TISSUES

Warm up tissues of the head and neck with gliding and light kneading strokes.

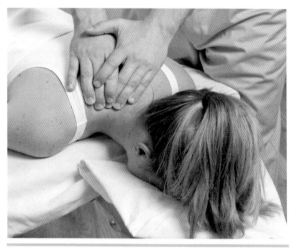

SEQUENCE 5-1 FIGURE 1

RESTRICTIONS AND TRIGGER POINTS

Address restrictions and trigger points in the upper trapezius.

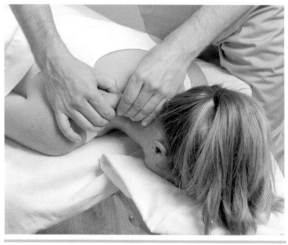

SEQUENCE 5-1 FIGURE 2

HEADACHES SEQUENCE

LEVATOR SCAPULAE

Address restrictions and trigger points in the levator scapulae using compression, lengthening strokes, and transverse friction.

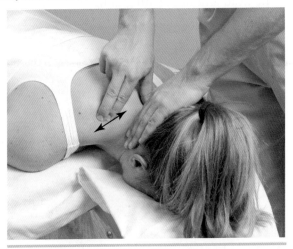

SEQUENCE 5-1 FIGURE 3

STERNOCLEIDOMASTOID

Address restrictions and trigger points in the SCM using stripping strokes and pincement. Transverse friction at attachment sites is beneficial.

CAUTION

The SCM borders the carotid artery and the jugular vein. Be aware of these structures and avoid.

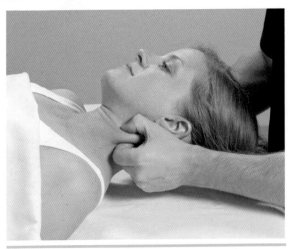

SEQUENCE 5-1 FIGURE 4

SCM, Sternocleidomastoid.

SCALENES

Address restrictions and trigger points using stripping strokes and compression.

CAUTION

The brachial plexus is found between the anterior and middle scalene muscles. Prolonged compression and misplacement of hands may aggravate this nerve.

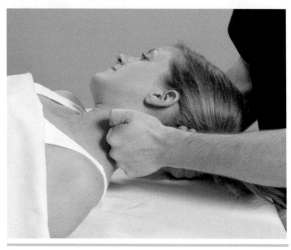

SEQUENCE 5-1 FIGURE 5

SUBOCCIPITAL GROUP

Compression and stripping strokes are effective with the suboccipitals. Use the weight of the head and neck as your resistance.

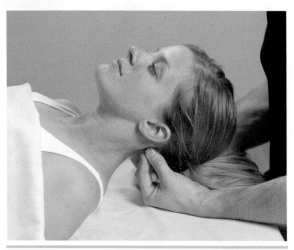

SEQUENCE 5-1 FIGURE 6

HEADACHES SEQUENCE

STRETCHING

Joint movements and stretching will help with cooling down the muscles.

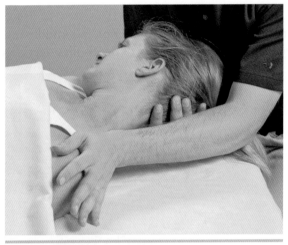

SEQUENCE 5-1 FIGURE 7

FACIAL MASSAGE

Finish with a facial massage and apply direct pressure to accupoints associated with headaches and sinus pressure.

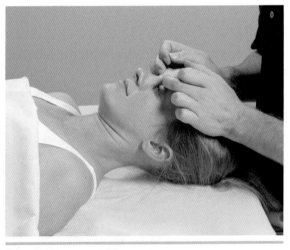

SEQUENCE 5-1 FIGURE 8

down and forward and backward, along with lateral motions. There is a lot of mobility in this joint that makes it prone to injury and repetitive use disorders. It also has a unique muscular feature in that the lateral pterygoid muscle connects directly to the articular disc of the TMJ.

Five muscles act to move the jaw and have a direct effect on the TMJ: temporalis, masseter, lateral and medial pterygoid, and the digastrics muscles. The temporalis muscle is primarily used to retract and elevate the mandible. It is constantly used when chewing and talking. The masseter muscle elevates and protracts the mandible, with the deep head aiding in retraction of the mandible. These two muscles are easily accessible and refer pain to the jaw and temple area (Figure 5-6).

The lateral pterygoid has the most direct influence on TMJ pain and dysfunction. This muscle attaches to the neck of the mandible and directly to the articular disk. It helps to protract and deviate the mandible to the opposite side. Because of the muscular and structural layout of the face, the best way to address this muscle is through intraoral techniques. The medial pterygoid helps to elevate, protract, and deviate the mandible. Although this muscle is best accessed through intraoral techniques, its attachment at the inner surface of the angle on the mandible can be palpated externally on the skin surface (Figure 5-7).

Because of the diverse causes of this disorder, it is best to consult with the client's physician to develop a plan. Repetitive use, consistent contraction, posture, and other factors can affect the function of these muscles resulting in generalized jaw pain, misalignment of the mandible, and even subluxation of the articulating cartilage. Even though a client may experience some of these symptoms, it is crucial that a physician confirm the diagnosis. In some cases, if the discomfort is due to wiring of the jaw, if there is abnormal growth and bone formations, or if the physician has a specific treatment plan for this client, the best approach is avoidance (Box 5-2) (Sequence 5-2).

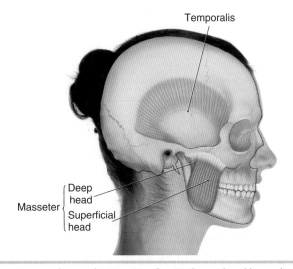

FIGURE 5-6 ■ Masseter and temporalis. (From Muscolino JE: *The muscle and bone palpation manual with trigger points, referral patterns, and stretching,* St Louis, 2009, Mosby.)

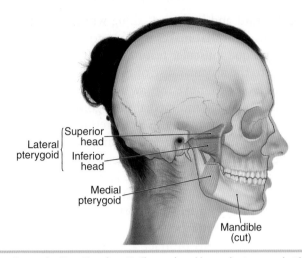

FIGURE 5-7 ■ Pterygoids. (From Muscolino, JE: *The muscle and bone palpation manual with trigger points, referral patterns, and stretching,* St Louis, 2009, Mosby.)

Box 5-2   SIGNS AND SYMPTOMS OF TEMPOROMANDIBULAR JOINT DISORDER

Clicking
Pain
Limited ROM (Range of Motion)
Muscular tension
Bruxism
Lock jaw
Difficulty opening the mouth
Pain when chewing or yawning
Headaches

TORTICOLLIS

Torticollis is the technical term for the condition commonly called "wryneck" or "a kink in the neck." It is characterized by a lateral tilt or contralateral rotation in the head. There are two main classifications of torticollis: congenital and spasmodic. **Congenital torticollis** is a genetic condition. It often occurs when the body develops only one SCM. In some infants, positioning of the head in utero may cause the SCM to be underdeveloped. In both instances, the condition may be corrected through early physical therapy intervention (Figure 5-8, p. 62).

Spasmodic torticollis (ST) can be due to an injury or trauma to the neck. The most common causes of ST are sleeping in a wrong or awkward position and injuries such as whiplash sustained in a car accident. The neck muscles become tight and protective, often unilaterally. The muscles that are affected are the SCM, scalenes, trapezius, and splenic muscles (Figure 5-9, p. 62).

SEQUENCE 5-2

WARM UP TISSUES OF THE HEAD AND NECK
Warm up the tissues surrounding the neck and head.

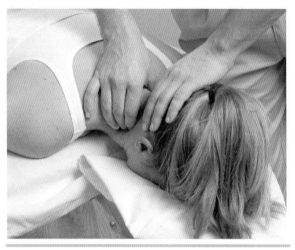

SEQUENCE 5-2 FIGURE 1

TEMPORALIS MUSCLE
Address any restrictions and trigger points of the temporalis muscle. Circular motions and stripping strokes from origin to insertion and transverse friction at the insertion are beneficial.

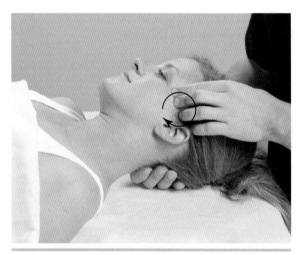

SEQUENCE 5-2 FIGURE 2

TEMPOROMANDIBULAR JOINT SEQUENCE

MASSETER MUSCLE

Use compression, stripping, and circular motions on the masseter to loosen and address restrictions.

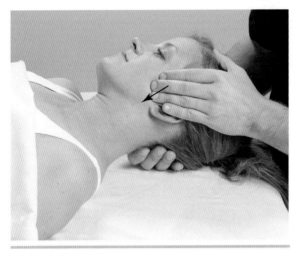

SEQUENCE 5-2 FIGURE 3

LATERAL PTERYGOID

Address trigger points on the lateral pterygoid. Have client open and close mouth to tolerance for active releases.

CAUTION

Trigger points in the lateral pterygoid can be extremely sensitive. The client will need to be in charge of the pressure to tolerance.

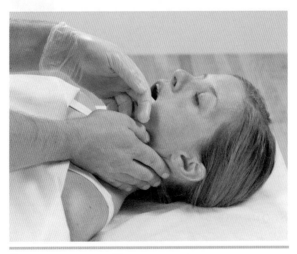

SEQUENCE 5-2 FIGURE 4

MEDIAL PTERYGOID

Address trigger points on the medial pterygoid. Have client open and close mouth to tolerance for active releases.

CAUTION

Trigger points in the lateral pterygoid can be extremely sensitive. The client will need to be in charge of the pressure to tolerance.

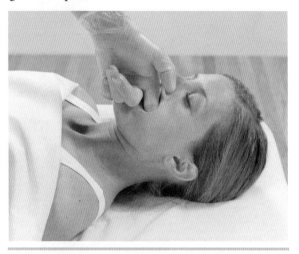

SEQUENCE 5-2 FIGURE 5

DISTRACTION AND MYOFASCIAL TECHNIQUES

Apply myofascial stretching and distraction to the TMJ.

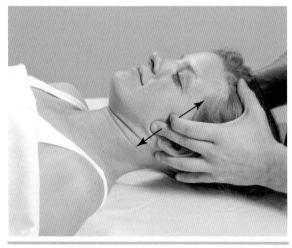

SEQUENCE 5-2 FIGURE 6

TMJ, Temporomandibular joint.

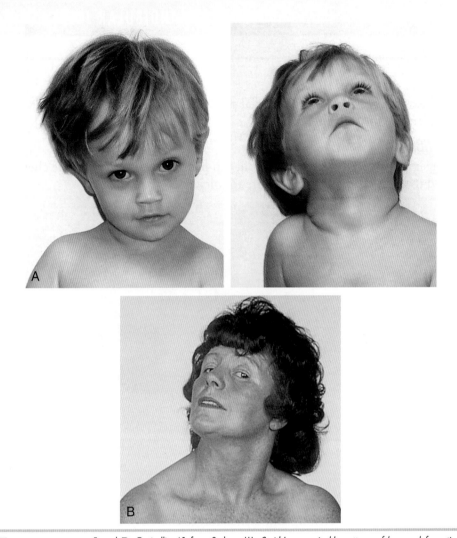

FIGURE 5-8 ■ **A** and **B,** Torticollis. (**A** from Graham JM: *Smith's recognizable patterns of human deformation,* Philadelphia, 2007, Saunders; **B** from Perkin GD: *Mosby's color atlas and text of neurology,* London, 1998, Mosby-Wolfe.)

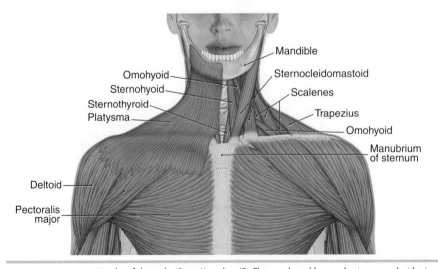

FIGURE 5-9 ■ Muscles of the neck. (From Muscolino JE: *The muscle and bone palpation manual with trigger points, referral patterns, and stretching,* St Louis, 2009, Mosby.)

It is important to remember that ST is due to an injury or trauma. ST may become a chronic condition; a thorough client history will help identify and get more information regarding this condition. Work in this area is contraindicated if the injury is less than 72 hours old. It is also important to look for signs of the inflammatory process. After the 3-day acute stage is over, these muscles tend to react well to general firm gliding. Moist heat helps warm the tissue and softens the connective tissues. Proprioceptive neuromuscular facilitation and stretching within tolerance is also beneficial. When working in this area, as you access the deeper layers of tissues, it is important to be aware of the underlying tissues and structures. Also be aware of the head positioning and severity of the ST. It may be uncomfortable for the client to be in a prone position for trapezius work. Most techniques are best applied in the supine or side-lying position. If you are going to use the side-lying positioning, be sure to support the head and neck to the client's comfort (Sequence 5-3).

WHIPLASH

Whiplash is an injury involving a sudden acceleration and deceleration, which causes hyperextension or hyperflexion of the head and neck. It is most often caused by motor vehicle accidents, sports injuries, high-speed rides like theme park rides and jet skis, or falls. Because of this sudden movement, whiplash usually involves trauma to the ligaments, muscles, joint capsules, or nervous system. Most injuries affect the area around the cervical vertebrae 4 and 5. Because of the severity of this type of injury, it is important to obtain a physician's release before you schedule a session. Fractured vertebrae can present the same symptoms as a whiplash injury and may go unnoticed without an x-ray examination. Many physicians first refer whiplash patients to physical therapists, as these injuries are severe and often require medications and advanced treatment options (Figure 5-10, p. 68).

The muscles that are prone to injury during whiplash are the SCM, scalenes, and splenius cervicis. Injuries may also occur to the supraspinous and intertransverse ligaments, which are the ligaments that traverse the spinous processes and transverse processes, respectively. The anterior and posterior longitudinal ligaments run along the anterior and posterior surface of the body of the vertebrae. Therapists cannot access these ligaments, making it difficult to identify; however, passive ROM can be used to assess whether damage has occurred to these ligaments. Other structures that can be injured, making this a severe injury, are the joint capsules, facet joints, intervertebral discs, and organs like the esophagus and larynx. It is important that physicians and therapists work together to develop a plan for massage intervention.

During the acute stage of whiplash injuries, massage is contraindicated. It is important to let the natural healing process and inflammation take care of itself. Once all other concerns like ruptured or herniated disks are ruled out, orthopedic or chiropractic adjustments and physical therapy usually proceed. These adjunct therapies work well to address the spinal alignment and injuries to the cervical vertebrae. If muscular spasms and pain continue, these adjustments may not have a long-term benefit. Taut and restricted muscles can pull the vertebrae

TORTICOLLIS SEQUENCE

SEQUENCE 5-3

WARM UP TISSUES OF THE NECK
Use effleurage and pétrissage to warm up the tissues of the neck.

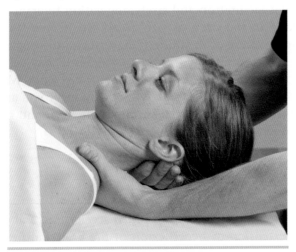

SEQUENCE 5-3 FIGURE 1

DEEP SPINAL MUSCLES
Strip the deep muscles along the lamina groove, moving from superior to inferior.

CAUTION
Go to client's tolerance with this technique; some clients may be sensitive in this area.

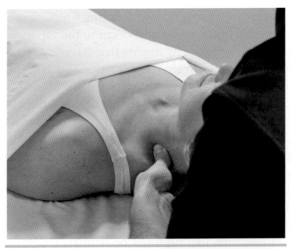

SEQUENCE 5-3 FIGURE 2

TORTICOLLIS SEQUENCE

STERNOCLEIDOMASTOID

Address restrictions and trigger points in the SCM using stripping strokes and pincement. Transverse friction at attachment sites is beneficial.

CAUTION

The SCM borders the carotid artery and the jugular vein. Be aware and avoid these structures.

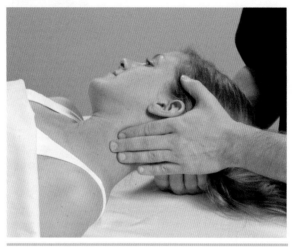

SEQUENCE 5-3 FIGURE 3

SCALENES

Address restrictions and trigger points using stripping strokes and compression.

CAUTION

The brachial plexus is found between the anterior and middle scalene muscles. Prolonged compression and misplacement of hands may aggravate this nerve.

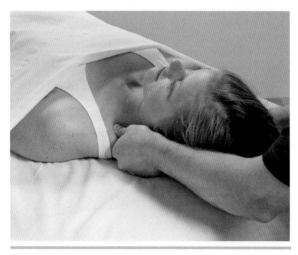

SEQUENCE 5-3 FIGURE 4

TORTICOLLIS SEQUENCE

ASSESS CERVICAL MOBILITY

Use joint movements to assess the mobility in the spine.

CAUTION

With torticollis, hypersensitivity may be present in multiple areas. Assess client conformability during these motions.

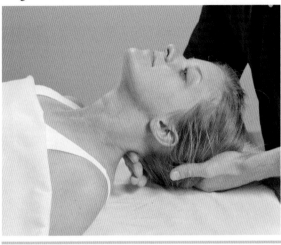

SEQUENCE 5-3 FIGURE 5

MANUAL HEAD (CERVICAL) TRACTION

Apply a light, consistent pull on the head supporting the neck for approximately 15-20 seconds.

CAUTION

It is important to maintain head position during this movement. Pull only until resistance is felt. *Do not* force this move.

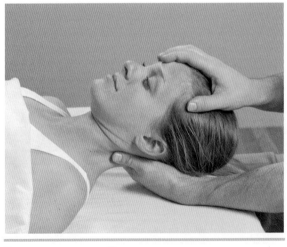

SEQUENCE 5-3 FIGURE 6

OCCIPITAL RELEASE

Perform a myofascial O-A release. Let the head fall naturally into your palms.

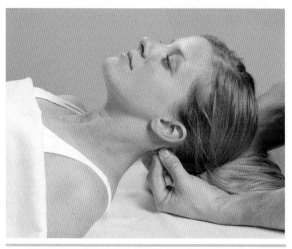

SEQUENCE 5-3 FIGURE 7

ENDING STROKES

Apply effleurage to help with circulation and neck stretches to end the session.

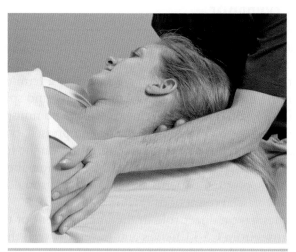

SEQUENCE 5-3 FIGURE 8

O-A, Occipito-Atlantal Joint; *SCM*, sternocleidomastoid.

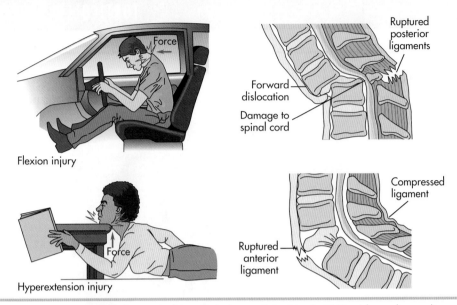

FIGURE 5-10 ■ Whiplash is a strain of the cervical spine, usually involving the C4-C5 vertebrae and surrounding musculature. Because of sudden backward and forward movements, damage can occur at the anterior or posterior aspects of the spine. (From Copstead-Kirkhorn: *Pathophysiology,* ed 4, St Louis, 2010, Saunders.)

out of alignment, creating ongoing symptoms. This is where the partnership of massage therapist and other health care practitioners like chiropractors, osteopaths, or orthopedic doctors work best for long-term results (Sequence 5-4).

THORACIC OUTLET SYNDROME

Thoracic outlet syndrome (TOS) is a group of disorders that result in compression of the neurovascular bundle, which consists of the brachial nerve plexus, axillary artery, and subclavian vein. *Thoracic outlet* is a term used to describe the area between the first rib, clavicle, coracoid process, and spine. There are three main classifications of TOS: neurogenic, vascular, and nonspecific. These classifications are based on the vessel that is being compressed, or where the sign and symptoms are present, but no specific compression can be found. The impingement of these vessels can be caused by anatomic anomalies such as a cervical rib or bone spurs, postural patterns such as retracted shoulders, trauma such as whiplash, or myofascial restrictions (Figure 5-11, p. 73).

The scalenes have a direct role in the impingement of the nerves. The brachial plexus arises from C5-T1 nerves and travels between the anterior and middle scalene. Taut bands or restrictions in these muscles can pinch these nerves, causing numbness or the "pins and needles" feeling down the arm. These muscles also elevate the first rib, which can pinch the subclavian vein and axillary artery, affecting circulation. The subclavian artery and vein traverse under the clavicle and under the pectoralis, which can also be a main contributor to impinging the blood vessels. Another muscle that plays a minor role in TOS is the subclavius. This muscle does not directly impinge any of the vessels; however, it does depress the clavicle and elevate the first rib, which can aid in narrowing the thoracic outlet where these vessels pass (Box 5-3, p. 73).

SEQUENCE 5-4

WARM UP TISSUES OF THE NECK

Use effleurage and pétrissage on the posterior cervical muscles from base to occiput.

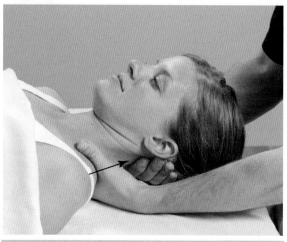

SEQUENCE 5-4 FIGURE 1

FRICTION SUBOCCIPITAL MUSCLES

Apply transverse friction to muscles inserting into the mastoid process and along the occipital ridge, including the suboccipital muscles.

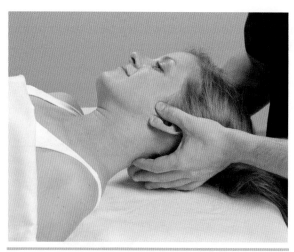

SEQUENCE 5-4 FIGURE 2

TRIGGER POINTS

Address any trigger points along the posterior and lateral cervical muscles.

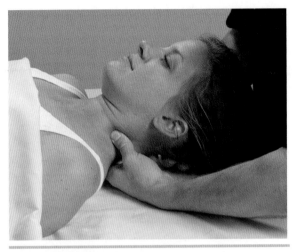

SEQUENCE 5-4 FIGURE 3

MUSCLE STRIPPING

Apply stripping strokes to the posterior and lateral muscles of the neck. Focus should be on the splenius and scalene muscles.

CAUTION

These may be sensitive because of injury. Keep clear communication with the client to stay within pain tolerance.

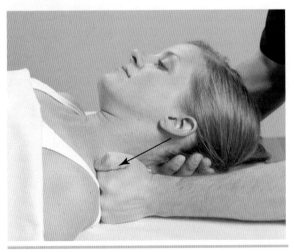

SEQUENCE 5-4 FIGURE 4

FRICTION TO LIGAMENTS

Apply transverse friction to the intertransverse ligaments.

CAUTION

Accessing and applying friction to these ligaments may be painful to the client. If it is painful, do not apply this technique.

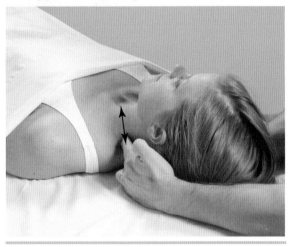

SEQUENCE 5-4 FIGURE 5

ANTERIOR CERVICAL MUSCLES

Address any trigger points found in the SCM and apply transverse friction to the insertion at the clavicle and sternum.

CAUTION

Use lighter pressure when working the anterior cervical muscles and work within tolerance. Be aware of endangerment sites.

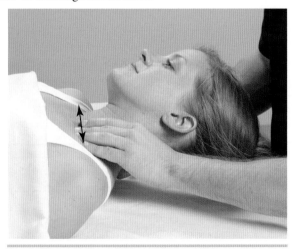

SEQUENCE 5-4 FIGURE 6

SCM, Sternocleidomastoid.

WHIPLASH SEQUENCE

JOINT MOVEMENTS
Finish the sequence with light joint movements and stretching.

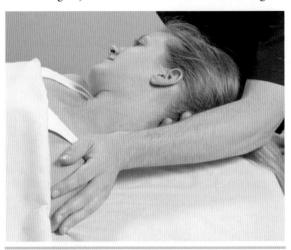

SEQUENCE 5-4 FIGURE 7

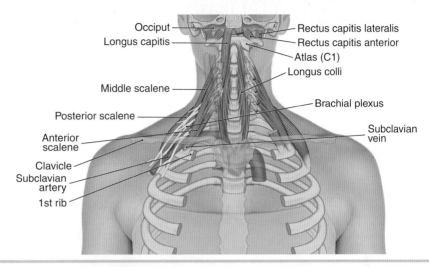

Occiput
Longus capitis
Rectus capitis lateralis
Rectus capitis anterior
Atlas (C1)
Longus colli
Middle scalene
Brachial plexus
Posterior scalene
Subclavian vein
Anterior scalene
Clavicle
Subclavian artery
1st rib

FIGURE 5-11 ■ Thoracic outlet. (From Muscolino JE: *The muscle and bone palpation manual with trigger points, referral patterns, and stretching,* St Louis, 2009, Mosby.)

Box 5-3 SIGNS AND SYMPTOMS OF THORACIC OUTLET SYNDROME

Shooting pains down the arm
Numbness or tingling
Weakness
Pain, mostly in the neck or top of shoulder
Fluid retention in the arm
Cold arm, hand, and fingers
Discoloration in the arm
Symptoms that worsen at night or when arm is over the head

Massage can work well with the muscular tension and weakness associated with TOS. The focus is to relax tight muscles while educating the client about postural habits that may be involved with these symptoms. Myofascial release techniques along with stripping and lengthening strokes work well to address muscular tightness. Structural approaches, stretching, and exercise can help improve posture and maintain structural alignment. If the root cause of the TOS is a cervical rib, bone spur, or other anatomic abnormality, massage should be given to help manage the discomfort and symptoms (Sequence 5-5).

THORACIC OUTLET SYNDROME SEQUENCE

SEQUENCE 5-5

WARM UP POSTERIOR TISSUES

Apply effleurage and pétrissage to posterior cervical muscles, trapezius, levators, and rhomboids.

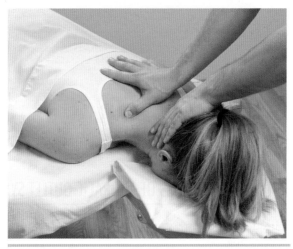

SEQUENCE 5-5 FIGURE 1

STRIPPING

Apply deep glides and stripping strokes to the levator, supraspinatus, and upper trapezius.

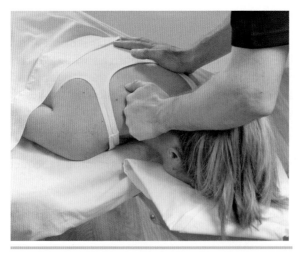

SEQUENCE 5-5 FIGURE 2

THORACIC OUTLET SYNDROME SEQUENCE

TRIGGER POINTS

Address trigger points found in posterior cervical muscles, trapezius, levators, and rhomboids.

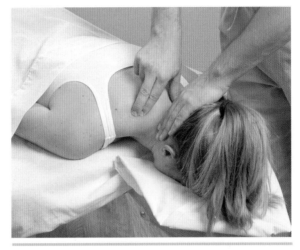

SEQUENCE 5-5 FIGURE 3

STRETCHING

Apply lateral cervical stretching. Rotate the head with each stretch to address different muscles.

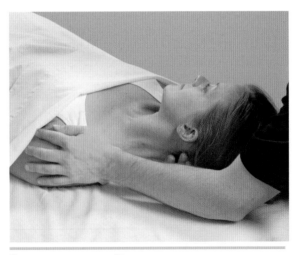

SEQUENCE 5-5 FIGURE 4

THORACIC OUTLET SYNDROME SEQUENCE

FRICTION SUBOCCIPITAL MUSCLES

Apply transverse friction to muscles inserting into the mastoid process and along the occipital ridge, including the suboccipital muscles.

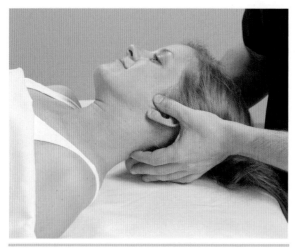

SEQUENCE 5-5 FIGURE 5

MUSCLE STRIPPING

Apply stripping strokes to the posterior and lateral muscles of the neck. Focus should be on the splenius and scalene muscles.

CAUTION

These muscles may be sensitive because of injury. Maintain clear communication with the client to stay within pain tolerance.

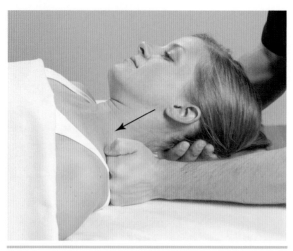

SEQUENCE 5-5 FIGURE 6

TRIGGER POINTS

Address trigger points found in scalene and splenius muscle groups.

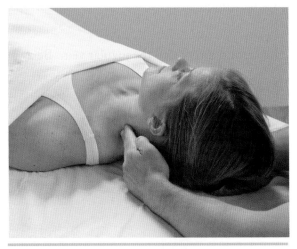

SEQUENCE 5–5 FIGURE 7

ANTERIOR CERVICAL MUSCLES

Address any trigger points found in the SCM and apply transverse friction to the insertion at the clavicle and sternum.

CAUTION

Use lighter pressure when working the anterior cervical muscles and work within tolerance. Be aware of endangerment sites.

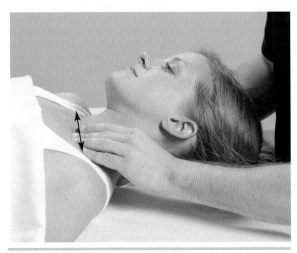

SEQUENCE 5–5 FIGURE 8

THORACIC OUTLET SYNDROME SEQUENCE

TRIGGER POINTS

Address restrictions and trigger points in the SCM using stripping strokes and pincement. Transverse friction at attachment sites is beneficial.

CAUTION

The SCM borders the carotid artery and the jugular vein. Be aware and avoid these structures.

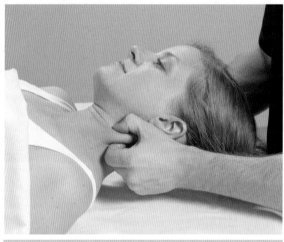

SEQUENCE 5–5 FIGURE 9

STRIPPING

Apply deep slides to the pectoralis major and compression to the pectoralis minor. Strokes should be lateral.

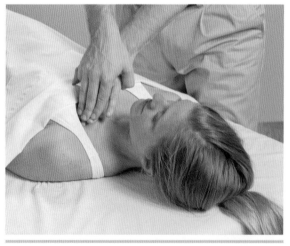

SEQUENCE 5–5 FIGURE 10

SCM, Sternocleidomastoid.

JOINT MOVEMENTS

End session with joint movements and stretching to neck and shoulder.

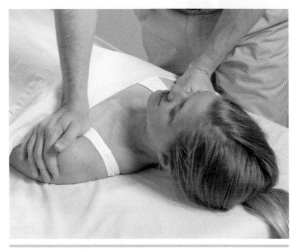

SEQUENCE 5-5 FIGURE 11

CHAPTER 6

SHOULDER

KEY TERMS

acromioclavicular (AC) joint
adhesive capsulitis
external rotators
glenohumeral joint
grade of injury
internal rotators
microtrauma
postisometric relaxation (PIR)
protection, rest, ice, compression,
  and elevation (PRICE) principle
rotator cuff
shoulder girdle
stages of adhesive capsulitis
sternoclavicular (SC) joint
winging scapula

OBJECTIVES

1 Understand the anatomy of the shoulder girdle.
2 Explain the joints of the shoulders and common injuries for these joints.
3 Apply bodywork techniques to specific injuries of the shoulder girdle.

The shoulder region is a complex area composed of muscles, bone tissues, and ligaments. It is a highly mobile region, which makes it more prone to injuries, repetitive-use trauma, muscle tears, and fatigue. The **shoulder girdle** is where the upper limb attaches to the torso through the sternoclavicular joint (Figure 6-1).

Most injuries to the shoulder girdle result from muscular, tendon, or ligament damage. Although prevalent in sports, shoulder injuries are becoming more common in our aging population. There are three main joints in the shoulder girdle and one articulation area. The **sternoclavicular (SC) joint** is the most stable and the strongest of these joints and is not injured often because of its strength. It is more common to break the clavicle or damage the **acromioclavicular (AC) joint** before damaging the SC joint. The AC joint connects the lateral head of the clavicle to the acromion process of the scapula. The AC joint has a weak joint capsule and is suspended in place by two ligaments. The **glenohumeral joint** is the ball and socket known as the *shoulder joint*. It has a shallow articulating surface held together through a joint capsule and several ligaments. This design makes the glenohumeral joint more susceptible to injuries. The scapulothoracic articulation is not a true joint, but it is

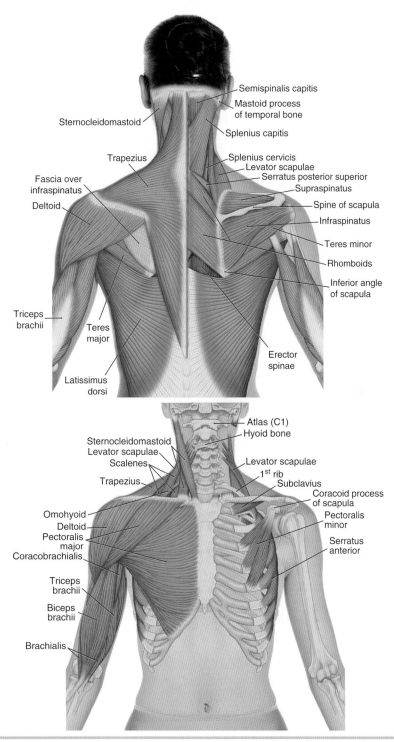

Semispinalis capitis
Mastoid process of temporal bone
Sternocleidomastoid
Splenius capitis
Trapezius
Splenius cervicis
Levator scapulae
Serratus posterior superior
Fascia over infraspinatus
Supraspinatus
Deltoid
Spine of scapula
Infraspinatus
Teres minor
Rhomboids
Inferior angle of scapula
Triceps brachii
Teres major
Erector spinae
Latissimus dorsi

Atlas (C1)
Hyoid bone
Sternocleidomastoid
Levator scapulae
Scalenes
Levator scapulae
1st rib
Trapezius
Subclavius
Coracoid process of scapula
Omohyoid
Deltoid
Pectoralis minor
Pectoralis major
Serratus anterior
Coracobrachialis
Triceps brachii
Biceps brachii
Brachialis

FIGURE 6-1 ■ Shoulder girdle. (Modified from Muscolino JE: *The muscle and bone palpation manual with trigger points, referral patterns, and stretching,* St Louis, 2009, Mosby.)

used to describe the movement between the scapula and the rib cage. This is an important area to study as it helps stabilize the shoulder while allowing for high mobility of the shoulder girdle.

ACROMIOCLAVICULAR JOINT INJURIES

The AC joint attaches the scapula to the clavicle. As stated previously, this is a weak gliding joint supported by two ligaments: the acromioclavicular ligament and the coracoclavicular ligament (Figure 6-2). There is a fibrous cartilage disk between the two bones in the majority of people. In some cases the acromion process fuses with the clavicle. Because of its structure, this joint is prone to injuries from bumps, falls, and other trauma. An AC joint injury is often referred to as a "separated shoulder." Trauma to this area is classified as a sprain as it usually affects the ligaments. AC sprains are described in four grades, or types, beginning with an overstretched ligament to a complete tear of both ligaments (Table 6-1).

When working with AC joint injuries it is important to remember that it is a ligamental injury. There are no muscles that act directly on this joint. The trapezius, pectoralis major, deltoid, and subclavius all share attachments on the

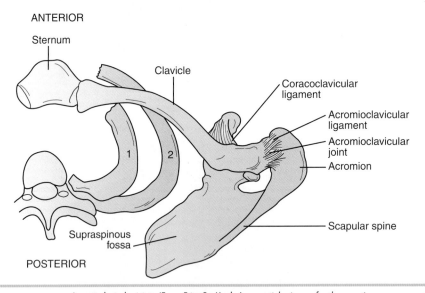

FIGURE 6-2 ■ Acromioclavicular joint. (From Fritz S: *Mosby's essential sciences for therapeutic massage: anatomy, physiology, biomechanics and pathology,* ed 3, St Louis, 2009, Mosby.)

Table 6-1 AC JOINT INJURY TYPES

Grade I	Sprain to both ligaments
Grade II	Tearing of the acromioclavicular ligament
Grade III	Tearing of the coracoclavicular ligament
Grade IV	Complete tearing of both ligaments with the clavicle being shifted out of alignment

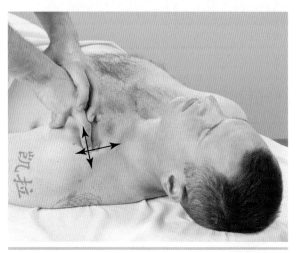

FIGURE 6-3 ■ Friction to the acromioclavicular joint.

clavicle and acromion process. Massage to these muscles is beneficial to keep these tissues pliable and free of adhesions or trigger points often created by the immobilization of the shoulder. As with all recent injuries the **protection, rest, ice, compression, and elevation (PRICE) principle** and no-hands approach are important for the first 48 to 72 hours. Depending on the **grade of injury**, the focus should be on relaxing the surrounding muscle tissues. When tolerable, friction to the joint helps with proper scar-tissue formation (Figure 6-3). With all grades of AC joint injuries, it is important to work with the physician and physical therapists to ensure the massage is helping the rehabilitation of the injury (Sequence 6-1).

ADHESIVE CAPSULITIS

More commonly known as "frozen shoulder," **adhesive capsulitis** is a disorder involving the joint capsule of the glenohumeral joint. The joint capsule starts to thicken and adhere to itself and the surrounding bones, causing pain and a loss of range of motion (Figure 6-4, p. 87). There is no known cause for this disorder, although it is commonly thought to start from a lesion, strain, or degeneration to the shoulder joint. It is also believed that people who have worn a sling or had the shoulder otherwise immobilized for several weeks are prone to frozen shoulder.

There are three **stages** to this disorder: the freezing phase, the frozen phase, and the thawing phase. During the freezing phase, the pain starts to build slowly and becomes more painful at night. The shoulder becomes inflamed and starts to lose its range of motion (ROM). This stage lasts approximately two to nine months, although it can be longer if an aggressive approach is applied, causing **microtrauma** and irritation to the area.

During the frozen phase the pain starts to diminish and the primary complaint becomes the lack of motion. This stage can last anywhere between 4 months and 1 year.

ACROMIOCLAVICULAR JOINT SEQUENCE

SEQUENCE 6-1

WARM UP SURROUNDING TISSUES

It is important to warm and loosen all surrounding tissues such as the trapezius, deltoid, rotator cuff muscles, and scalenes.

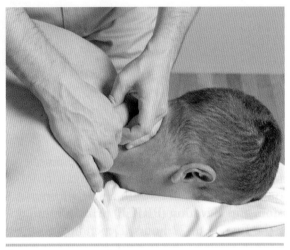

SEQUENCE 6-1 FIGURE 1

STRIPPING TO THE SUPERIOR MUSCLES

Start superior and strip the upper trapezius from the nuchal line to the AC joint. Strip the scalenes in the same manner.

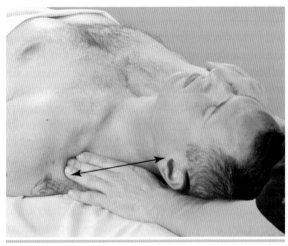

SEQUENCE 6-1 FIGURE 2

KNEADING THE DELTOID

Knead and broaden the deltoid muscle working distally to proximally. Focus on cross-fiber strokes along the proximal attachment.

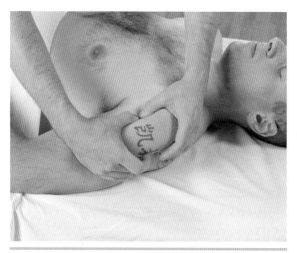

SEQUENCE 6–1 FIGURE 3

FRICTION THE AC JOINT

Apply multidirectional friction around the AC joint and the acromioclavicular ligament.

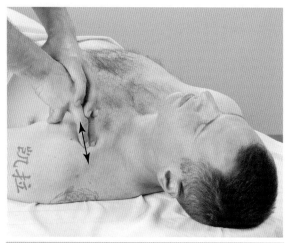

SEQUENCE 6–1 FIGURE 4

AC, Acromioclavicular.

ACROMIOCLAVICULAR JOINT SEQUENCE

WORK THE SUBCLAVICULAR AREA

Apply cross-fiber friction to the coracoclavicular ligament, and strip the subclavius muscle.

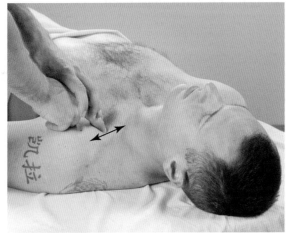

SEQUENCE 6-1 FIGURE 5

COOL DOWN TISSUES

Administer effleurage and pétrissage techniques to encourage circulation and as a transition to the next body segment.

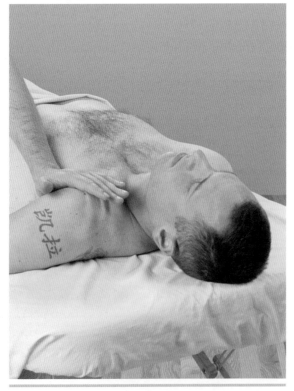

SEQUENCE 6-1 FIGURE 6

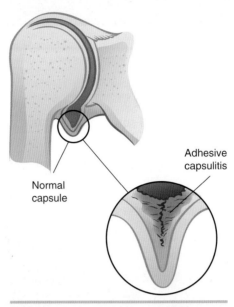

FIGURE 6-4 ■ Adhesive capsulitis. (From Shankman GA, et al: *Fundamental orthopedic management for the physical therapy assistant,* ed 2, Philadelphia, 2004, Mosby.)

During the thawing stage the pain continues to diminish and ROM gradually increases. Some therapists and physicians say that the time spent in the first two stages equals the time spent in the third stage. Others say the adhesive capsulitis can heal itself in approximately 2 years. Some studies have shown that people can experience minor complaints for many years after the condition.

Adhesive capsulitis reacts to a variety of therapeutic approaches. During the freezing stage physicians often prescribe antiinflammatory medicine to aid with the swelling and physical therapy to help with ROM. Massage therapy during this stage should focus on stress and pain reduction. It is important to work the associated muscles such as the rotator muscles, deltoid, and latissimus dorsi to help prevent trigger-point formation and hypertonicity. Passive joint movement within the clients' pain threshold has also shown benefits. It is important to avoid aggressive approaches. During the frozen stage focus should be on the reduction of hypertonic muscles and any trigger points that may have formed. In this stage, joint mobilizations can become more active and **postisometric relaxation (PIR)** techniques can be beneficial. Myofascial stretching to remove fascial adhesions is also performed in this stage (Sequence 6-2).

ROTATOR CUFF INJURIES

Rotator cuff injuries are becoming more common. As discussed earlier, the glenohumeral joint is not a stable or well-protected joint because of its bone structure. The glenoid fossa is shallow, requiring muscles, joint capsule, ligaments, and tendons to support the joint and maintain its position. Four main muscles compose the rotator cuff and help hold the head of the humerus to the glenoid fossa. The supraspinatus attaches to the greater tubercle of the humerus, initiating

Text continued on p. 92

ADHESIVE CAPSULITIS SEQUENCE

SEQUENCE 6-2

WARM UP SURROUNDING TISSUES

It is important to warm and loosen all surrounding tissues such as the latissimus dorsi, deltoid, rotator cuff muscles, and rhomboids.

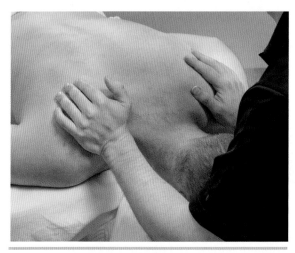

SEQUENCE 6-2 FIGURE 1

RANGE OF MOTION

Apply slight traction supporting the wrist and elbow. Slowly walk around the client to his or her limitations, maintaining the traction. Keep within the client's pain threshold; do not force the tissues.

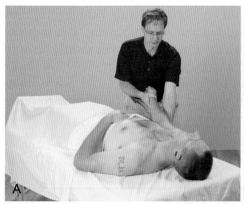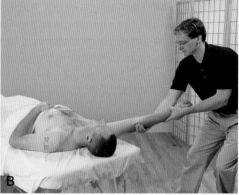

SEQUENCE 6-2 FIGURE 2A,B

MYOFASCIAL RELEASES

Hold the traction of the shoulder joint focusing on the fascia of the joint capsule. Follow the fascial releases as they occur.

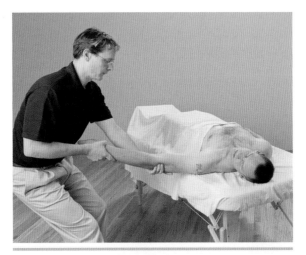

SEQUENCE 6-2 FIGURE 3

BROADENING AND STRIPPING OF THE LATISSIMUS DORSI

Flex the shoulder to tolerance and address the latissimus dorsi muscle.

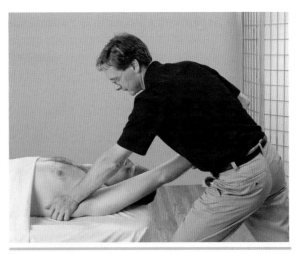

SEQUENCE 6-2 FIGURE 4

ADHESIVE CAPSULITIS SEQUENCE

DEEP FASCIAL WORK AROUND THE JOINT CAPSULE

Working into the joint capsule area needs to be performed *slowly and within tolerance.*

CAUTION

Be cautious of the vessels, nerves, and structures of the axillary area. *May be too aggressive for the freezing and frozen stages.*

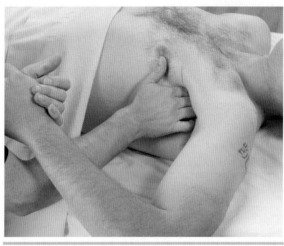

SEQUENCE 6-2 FIGURE 5

ADDRESS TRIGGER POINTS

Address any trigger points or hypertonic muscles in the surrounding tissues.

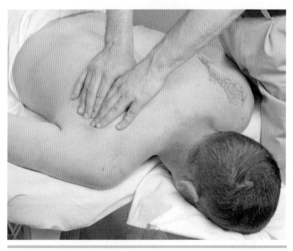

SEQUENCE 6-2 FIGURE 6

ADHESIVE CAPSULITIS SEQUENCE

LIGHT STRETCHING

Apply light stretching for the shoulder.

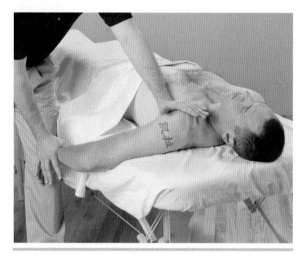

SEQUENCE 6-2 FIGURE 7

FINISH WITH EFFLEURAGE

Effleurage and circulation strokes are important at the end of intense work.

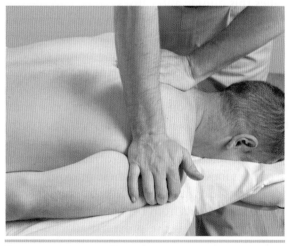

SEQUENCE 6-2 FIGURE 8

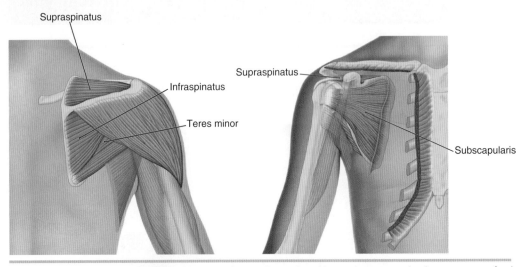

Supraspinatus

Infraspinatus

Supraspinatus

Teres minor

Subscapularis

FIGURE 6-5 ■ Rotator cuff. (Modified from Muscolino JE: *The muscle and bone palpation manual with trigger points, referral patterns, and stretching*, St Louis, 2009, Mosby.)

shoulder abduction. The infraspinatus and teres minor attach to the greater tubercle of the humerus producing external (lateral) rotation. The subscapularis attaches to the lesser tubercle as an internal (medial) rotator (Figure 6-5).

INTERNAL ROTATORS

The subscapularis lies between the rib cage and the scapula. Every time we reach into the back seat to get an object and bring it to the front seat, we are internally rotating the shoulder. When throwing a ball like a pitcher, quarterback, or soccer goalie, this muscle is engaged. Activities of daily living put more stress on **internal rotators** than on external rotators. Repetitive trauma and overuse fatigues this muscle and causes damage to the ligaments and tendons.

Therapists take multiple approaches to access the subscapularis muscle. In the prone position, it is common practice to place the client's wrist and forearm on his or her back. This position lifts the vertebral border of the scapula away from the ribcage, allowing access to the subscapularis proximal attachment site. Although this position is advantageous for the therapist, it is not always comfortable for the client (Figure 6-6). This position requires that the external rotators lengthen, which increases the pull at their distal attachment site. Too much pressure is placed on the anterior capsule and may cause more damage to the joint and surrounding structures. Many people may have microtrauma and adhesions in their shoulders because of their lifestyle and jobs; these microtraumas and adhesions shorten these muscles and create trigger points. Repetitive trauma in the shoulder may prevent many older adult clients from being placed in this position.

Another option to access the proximal attachment of the subscapularis is to manually lift the scapula away from the ribcage. This can be achieved in the prone position by supporting the anterior shoulder in the palm of your hand and grabbing the scapula with your other hand. It is helpful to perform some joint movements prior to trying to lift the scapula. This aids the client in relaxing the shoulder and warms the deep fascia and joint capsule. As you lift the shoulder, support the scapula with your other hand, then slide your fingers under the scapula to the subscapularis. It is crucial that you address the needs of the

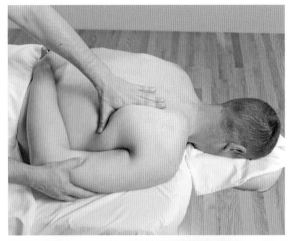

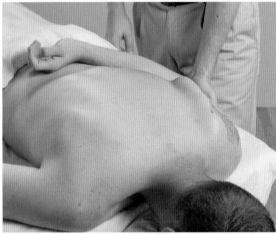

FIGURE 6-6 ■ **Winging**: arm behind the back. **Caution:** This position increases pressure on the anterior capsule and can be uncomfortable. *Not recommended.*

trapezius and the rhomboids first, or you will not be able to penetrate these muscles. This can also be performed in the side-lying position (Figure 6-7).

The supine position is the best position to access the belly of the subscapularis. This involves working in the axillary area, so be careful of vessels and work slowly. Abduct the shoulder to open the armpit. Place your fingers approximately halfway between the anterior and posterior surfaces of the body against the ribs. Follow the ribs in a posterior-superior direction. You will need to get under the latissimus dorsi and teres muscles. Externally rotate the shoulder to "pop" this muscle out to confirm that you are in the correct area. Effective techniques in this position include pin and stretch and slow stripping strokes (Figure 6-8).

This supine position is also a good position to access the distal attachment site of the subscapularis. Place the client's hands on his or her stomach and palpate the shoulder to find the lesser tubercle of the humerus and the coracoid process of the scapula. Place your fingers approximately halfway between these two landmarks. Apply pressure downward, laterally, and slightly inferiorly to access the medial border of the lesser tubercle. Cross-fiber friction to

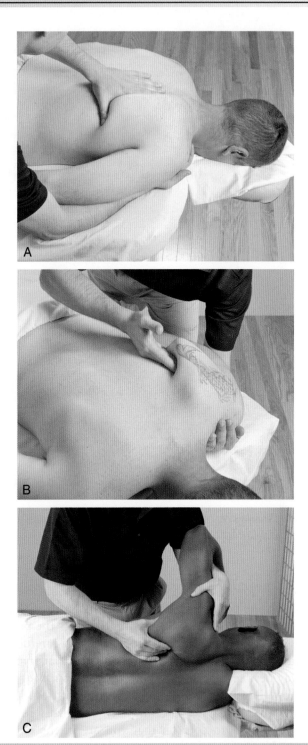

FIGURE 6-7 ■ Lifting of the scapula. **A & B,** Supported shoulder. Support the shoulder with one hand and move into a position where the scapula is elevated from rib cage. This position allows for more comfort and access to underlying tissues. **C,** Side-lying. Positioning in the side-lying posture allows for winging of the scapula.

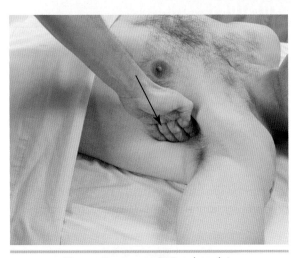

FIGURE 6-8 ■ Supine subscapularis.

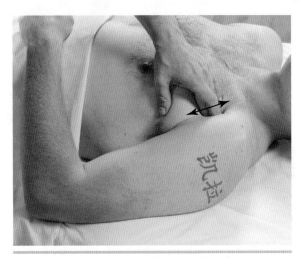

FIGURE 6-9 ■ Frictioning subscapularis.

the subscapularis tendon is effective to help break the adhesions of this muscle (Figure 6-9).

The subscapularis is not the only muscle involved in internal rotation of the shoulder. The latissimus dorsi, anterior deltoid, and teres major also play a role in internal rotation. If the subscapularis becomes torn or injured, these muscles compensate, which can make them more prone to injury and fatigue (Sequence 6-3).

EXTERNAL ROTATORS

External rotator cuff injuries are not as common as internal rotator injuries and they are more difficult to assess. The external rotator cuff muscles that come together to form the rotator cuff are the supraspinatus, infraspinatus, and teres minor. Severe injuries to the external rotators usually affect the tendon, which makes this injury difficult to diagnose. Passive, active, and resistive ROM can help isolate sore or injured muscles (Figure 6-10, p. 100).

INTERNAL ROTATORS SEQUENCE

SEQUENCE 6-3

WARM UP TISSUES

Warm up tissues with compression, muscle squeezing, and range-of-motion techniques.

CAUTION

The axillary area can be sensitive for many people and gliding strokes may induce a tickling feeling; compression and muscle squeezing can aid in avoiding this feeling.

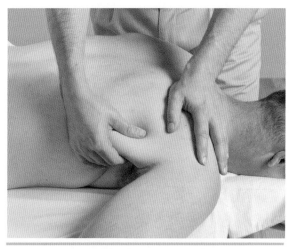

SEQUENCE 6–3 FIGURE 1

ADDRESS HYPERTONIC MUSCLES AND TRIGGER POINTS

Address trigger points found in latissimus dorsi, subscapularis, and anterior deltoids.

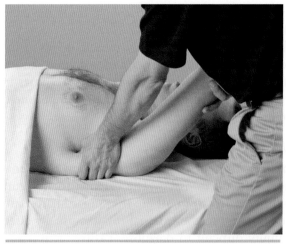

SEQUENCE 6–3 FIGURE 2

INTERNAL ROTATORS SEQUENCE

WORK THE SUBSCAPULARIS BELLY
Use slow compressive and deep strokes.

CAUTION
Be cautious of vessels and structures in the area. Strokes need to be slow and controlled.

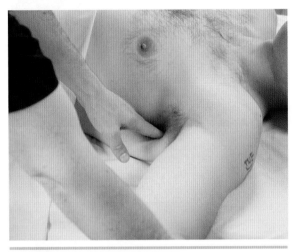

SEQUENCE 6-3 FIGURE 3

RANGE OF MOTION
Apply a small amount of traction throughout this series of movements. Let the shoulder move naturally and pause at any restriction felt. Focus on the fascial melting and unwinding during this movement.

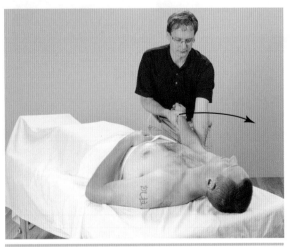

SEQUENCE 6-3 FIGURE 4A

INTERNAL ROTATORS SEQUENCE

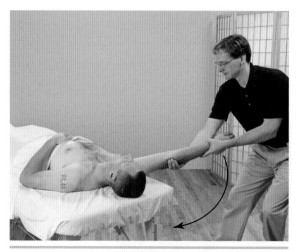

Sequence 6-3 Figure 4B

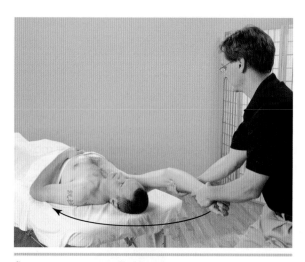

Sequence 6-3 Figure 4C

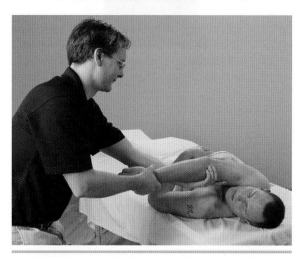

SEQUENCE 6–3 FIGURE 4D

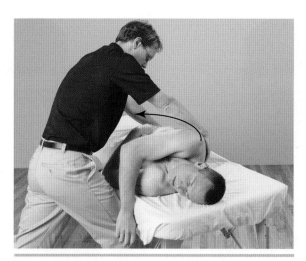

SEQUENCE 6–3 FIGURE 4E

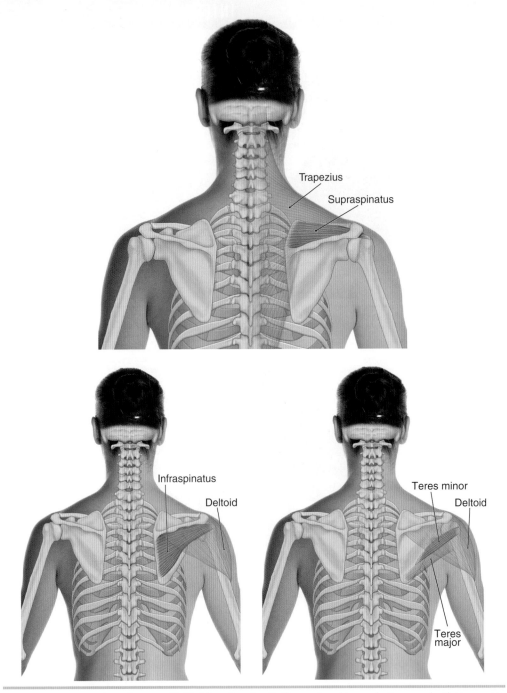

FIGURE 6-10 ■ External rotators. (Modified from Muscolino JE: *The muscle and bone palpation manual with trigger points, referral patterns, and stretching,* St Louis, 2009, Mosby.)

The supraspinatus is tucked into the supraspinous fossa of the scapula and under the trapezius. Its distal attachment point is on the superior aspect of the greater tubercle of the humerus. As this muscle reveals itself from under the acromion process, it provides the therapist with an access point to apply cross-fiber friction to the tendon. The supraspinatus plays two roles in the movement of the shoulder, to initiate shoulder abduction and to aid in external rotation. It also plays a key role in stabilizing the humerus to the glenoid fossa.

The infraspinatus, although superficial, does not get the attention it deserves. The infraspinatus is the largest of the external rotators and it is common for this muscle to be sensitive and tender. The infraspinatus has three common areas of hypersensitivity, and its distal attachment point can be frictioned on the border of the greater tubercle of the humerus.

The teres minor is also easily accessed in the axillary area. It originates on the axial border of the scapula and inserts into the greater tubercle of the humerus. A great technique to use with the teres minor is pincement.

Shoulder injuries are commonplace not only in athletes, but also with the process of aging. Approximately 60% of doctor visits for shoulder pain are due to rotator cuff injuries. Public education should focus on knowledge of common injuries, their frequency and causes, and injury prevention. At the onset of shoulder pain, stretching and exercise are two components to promote health and rehabilitation of the injury.

CHAPTER 7

ARM AND HAND

KEY TERMS

annular ligament
axillary nerve
brachial plexus
carpal tunnel
carpal tunnel syndrome
cervical nerve plexus
distal ulnar tunnel
distraction
fascia
fibrous joint capsule
flexor retinaculum
Guyon canal
humeroradial joint
humeroulnar joint
impingement
lateral collateral (radial) ligament
medial collateral (ulnar) ligament
median nerve
musculocutaneous nerve
musculotendinous
pronator teres syndrome
proximal radioulnar joint
proximal ulnar (cubital) tunnel
radial nerve
repetitive motions
traction
transverse carpal ligament
tendonitis
tendinosis
tunnel
ulnar nerve

OBJECTIVES

1   Understand the musculoskeletal design of the arm.

2   Explain the design of the elbow joint.

3   List and describe the ligament of the elbow joint.

4   Describe and identify common locations of nerve impingements in the elbow.

5   List and describe the nerves of the arm.

6   Explain the differences between tendonitis and tendinosis.

7   Demonstrate massage applications for arm massage.

8   Demonstrate techniques to treat carpal tunnel syndrome.

The muscles and joints located in the arm and hand make this a complex region. This chapter focuses on common **musculotendinous** complaints surrounding the elbow and wrist. These muscles can become fatigued, tighten, and cause pain because of **repetitive motions** and overuse.

Although classified as a hinge joint, the elbow is unique in that it has three articulations located within one joint capsule. Both the **humeroradial** and the **humeroulnar joints** work together to allow flexion and extension of the forearm. The **proximal radioulnar joint** allows for pronation and supination of the wrist (Figure 7-1).

The elbow has a complex design of ligaments to help support and protect the joint consisting of the three bones and three articulation structures. These ligaments are the **medial collateral (ulnar) ligament**, the **lateral collateral (radial) ligament**, the **annular ligament**, and the **fibrous joint capsule** (Figure 7-2).

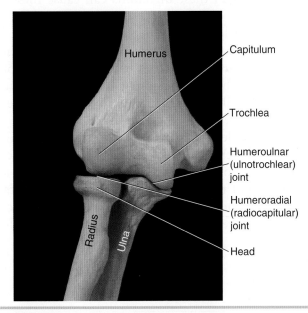

FIGURE 7-1 ▦ Elbow joint. (From Muscolino JE: *Kinesiology: the skeletal system and muscle function,* ed 2, St Louis, 2011, Mosby.)

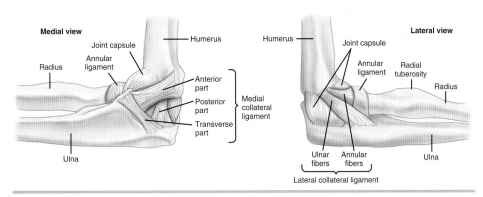

FIGURE 7-2 ▦ Elbow ligaments. (From Muscolino JE: *Kinesiology: the skeletal system and muscle function,* ed 2, St Louis, 2011, Mosby.)

The lateral and medial collateral ligaments help hold the ulna and the humerus bones together. These ligaments help protect the side-to-side movement or lateral stability of the elbow. The lateral collateral ligament has one proximal attachment site and two distal attachments, the ulna and the annular ligament. The medial collateral ligament has three sections with fibers running in different directions. The anterior portion attaches the lateral epicondyle to the coronoid process of the ulna. The posterior portion attaches the lateral epicondyle to the olecranon process of the ulna. The transverse fibers run from the distal attachment point of the anterior fibers across the trochlear notch to the attachment of the posterior fibers. Abduction or adduction at the elbow can cause stress to these ligaments. Repetitive motions or sudden movements in these directions can cause these ligaments to tear or rupture.

The radius is held securely in place by the annular ligament. This band attaches from the posterior aspect of the radial notch of the ulna, wraps around the neck of the radius, and attaches back into the anterior aspect of the radial notch of the ulna. This design allows for the flexion and extension to occur at the elbow but also allows for the radius to rotate over the ulna to pronate and supinate the forearm.

The main muscles that directly move the elbow joint are the bicep brachii, brachialis, brachioradialis, triceps brachii, and anconeus. The muscles that act on the radioulnar joints are the pronator teres and supinator at the proximal joint and the pronator quadratus at the distal joint. The flexors and extensors of the forearm also play minor roles to aid in flexion and extension of the forearm, but have a bigger role with flexion and extension of the wrist.

NERVE IMPINGEMENTS

The **brachial plexus** originates from the lower half of the **cervical nerve plexus** (C5-T1). It divides into five nerves at the shoulder traveling through the arm: the **ulnar**, **median**, **radial**, **axillary**, and **musculocutaneous** nerves. Because of the structure and muscles in the elbow region and the superficial location of some of these nerves, they are more prone to injuries from compression and impacts. The ulnar, median, and radial nerves cross the elbow joint with the protection of **tunnels**, **fascia**, muscles, and the bones, and are commonly impinged or injured (Figure 7-3).

ULNAR NERVE

The ulnar nerve passes through two ulnar tunnels. The **proximal ulnar (cubital) tunnel** can be found between the distal aspect of the medial condyle of the humerus and the olecranon process of the ulna. This is the nerve that most people refer to as the "funny bone." Most people have hit this nerve, creating the unmistakable "pins and needles" feeling down the forearm into the pinkie and the medial half of the ring finger. The **distal ulnar tunnel**, or **Guyon canal**, is located in the wrist between the pisiform bone and the hook of the hamate.

RADIAL NERVE

The radial nerve travels through the radial tunnel, which is situated under the supinator muscle. Tightness in this muscle can compress the radial nerve, creating pain near the elbow, forearm weakness and discomfort, and pain when extending the elbow and pronating the forearm. This **impingement** can be mistaken for lateral epicondylitis as they have similar symptoms.

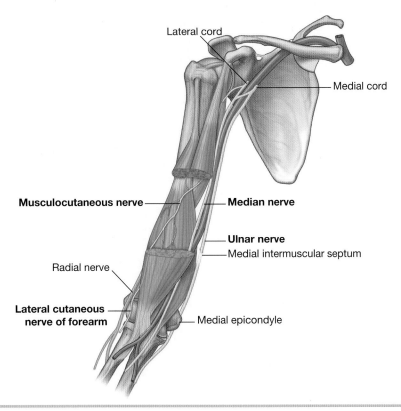

Lateral cord

Medial cord

Musculocutaneous nerve

Median nerve

Ulnar nerve

Medial intermuscular septum

Radial nerve

Lateral cutaneous
nerve of forearm

Medial epicondyle

FIGURE 7-3 ■ Nerves of the arm. (From Drake et al: *Gray's anatomy for students,* ed 2, New York, 2009, Churchill Livingstone.)

MEDIAN NERVE

The median nerve is most well known for its involvement and association with carpal tunnel syndrome. It is a branch of the brachial plexus and at the elbow passes between the two heads of the pronator teres muscle. The median nerve is the only nerve that passes through the carpal tunnel at the wrist. The median nerve feeds the lateral or radial aspect of the palm, digits 1-3, and the radial half of digit 4.

Common impingement locations for the median nerve occur with the pronator teres and at the carpal tunnel. It can be difficult to differentiate between impingements of the median nerve and the radial nerve. When in doubt, refer the client to a physician for further testing.

MUSCLES OF THE ARM

SUPINATOR

To access the supinator muscle you need to loosen the extensor group focusing on the extensor carpi radialis brevis and the extensor digitorum. Move the elbow into a position at approximately 90 degrees because this position helps

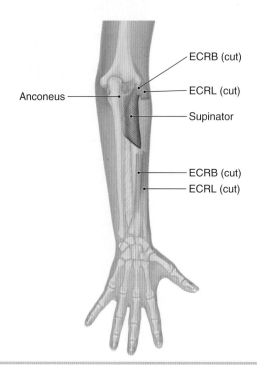

Anconeus

ECRB (cut)

ECRL (cut)

Supinator

ECRB (cut)

ECRL (cut)

FIGURE 7-4 ▪ Supinator. (From Muscolino JE: *The muscle and bone palpation manual with trigger points, referral patterns, and stretching,* St Louis, 2009, Mosby.)

shorten and relax the extensor group. Starting from the proximal forearm, find the brachioradialis. Moving laterally, the next muscle is the extensor carpi radialis longus and brevis. You will note a valley between the carpi radialis and the extensor digitorum. This valley is the easiest access point for the supinator muscle (Figure 7-4).

PRONATOR TERES

The pronator teres muscle is a bicep muscle having two heads. Its proximal attachments, or origins, are at the medial epicondyle of the humerus and the coronoid process of the ulna. These two heads merge together and attach to the lateral surface of the radius. The pronator teres's main function is to pronate the forearm and it also plays a role in flexion of the elbow. This muscle can be involved in a nerve impingement of the median nerve known as **pronator teres syndrome**. Pronator teres syndrome is often mistaken for carpal tunnel syndrome because they have similar signs and symptoms, including numbness in the first three digits. Pronator teres syndrome shows weakness specifically in the index finger, which affects the pincer movement and strength (Figure 7-5).

To access the pronator teres muscle it is important to work through the superficial layers of the fascia, the flexor carpi radialis and the brachioradialis. The pronator teres is found between these two muscles on the anterior surface of the forearm. It is a superficial muscle and it forms the distal medial border of the antecubital fossa endangerment site. Remember to use caution when

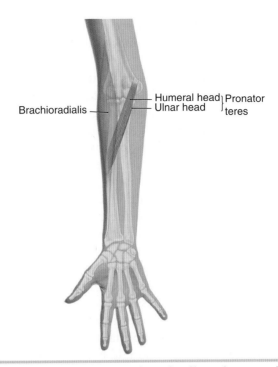

FIGURE 7-5 ■ Pronator teres. (From Muscolino JE: *The muscle and bone palpation manual with trigger points, referral patterns, and stretching,* St Louis, 2009, Mosby.)

working this muscle. Static digital compression to work the trigger points, cross-fiber friction, and active movements are effective techniques.

EPICONDYLITIS: TENDONITIS OR TENDINOSIS

New research regarding fascia and fascial disorders makes it necessary to revisit our approach to epicondylitis. The term *epicondylitis* roughly translates into "the swelling of the epicondyles." This disorder can be more accurately described as a tendonitis or tendinosis of the tendons attaching to the epicondyle. Lateral epicondylitis of the humerus involves the extensor tendons of the forearm, and medial epicondylitis of the humerus affects the flexor tendons of the wrist.

A paradigm shift in our approach starts with thinking about whether this disorder is a true tendonitis or a tendinosis. **Tendonitis** is the inflammation of the tendon caused by injury or trauma of some sort. This inflammation is associated with redness, heat, swelling, and pain. Most of the clients who come across our tables do not present these signs, and when they do, we approach them with the basic first aid for a new injury. Protection, rest, ice, compression, and elevation is the only treatment that should be used for new or acute injuries.

Tendinosis refers to the degradation of the fibers and cells of the tendon. This is the result of chronic stress, repetitive motions, or overuse activities that cause damage to the collagen and fibers of the tendon. This may more accurately define the disorder we see in our clients. Tendinosis does not present the redness or swelling of tendonitis, but it may also cause discomfort and pain.

With this understanding of *-osis* versus *-itis,* our approach to lateral epicondylitis, or tennis elbow, should shift. Lateral epicondylitis is usually caused by degradation of the extensor radialis longus. As new fibrous tissues are formed as scar tissue, the traditional approach has been to administer transverse friction to realign the collagen fibers to promote healthy tissue growth. The error of this thought process is twofold. The first error is the belief that performing one directional friction to a matrix composed of multidirectional fibers is as effective as administering multidirectional friction. The second and more important error is the belief that the tendon will be able to heal and repair itself when the muscle belly and fascia still have adhesions and contractions within their tissues.

The first step in addressing clients with epicondylitis is to address the needs of the muscles involved and return them to their normal resting length. Relaxing the muscle and addressing the hypercontractions or hyperirritability, helps alleviate some of the tension that is being applied to the tendon. Working through the layers is important for all forms of elbow pain. Skin rolling and myofascial techniques should be used first. This can be followed with general kneading to the forearm muscles. Stripping or broadening strokes, followed by multidirectional friction, have shown positive results. Most importantly, stretching of the tight, shortened muscles and strengthening for the long, weak muscles should be performed to bring the muscles back into balance. Ice massage around the epicondyle has also shown positive effects and can help control the inflammation therapists often create when working with epicondylitis (Sequence 7-1).

CARPAL TUNNEL SYNDROME

Carpal tunnel syndrome is a disorder that has been the subject of some controversy surrounding accurate diagnosis. The median nerve and flexor tendons traverse through this **carpal tunnel**, which is located in the wrist under the **transverse carpal ligament**, or **flexor retinaculum**, and anterior to the carpal bones. True carpal tunnel syndrome results in a pinching of the median nerve in this area. This impingement can be the result of an increase in fluids, inflammation, or scar tissue, which decreases the diameter of the tunnel. Characteristics of this disorder are numbness; tingling; and loss of strength in the thumb, index, and middle fingers, and half of the ring finger. Many cases of carpal tunnel syndrome result in surgical scraping to remove scar tissue and increase the opening to alleviate the pressure on the median nerve (Figure 7-6, p. 112).

Some of the controversy surrounding carpal tunnel syndrome concerns other locations of impingement of this nerve. Impingements in the cervical region, shoulder, and elbow may create symptoms similar to those of carpal tunnel syndrome. Testing to cancel out a brachial plexus impingement or radial nerve impingement is important. Often these tests are advanced for the

ELBOW TECHNIQUES SEQUENCE

SEQUENCE 7-1

WARM UP

Use pétrissage to warm up the tissues of the arm and forearm. Use broadening strokes and deep slides from distal to proximal on the forearm to loosen the tissue.

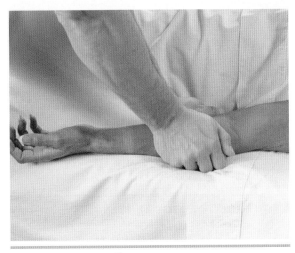

SEQUENCE 7-1 FIGURE 1

FOREARM MUSCLES

Use pincer techniques to address trigger points in the extensor muscles. Use passive motions by flexing and extending the wrist. Use deep longitudinal stripping strokes to break adhesions.

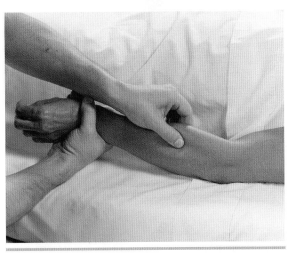

SEQUENCE 7-1 FIGURE 2

ELBOW TECHNIQUES SEQUENCE

FLEXOR AND EXTENSOR TENDON

Apply deep multidirectional friction to the common extensor and flexor tendons.

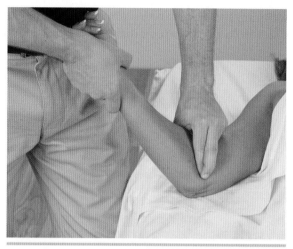

SEQUENCE 7-1 FIGURE 3

PRONATOR TERES

Apply deep longitudinal slides to the pronator teres. Compress the pronator teres and move the hand from pronation to supination.

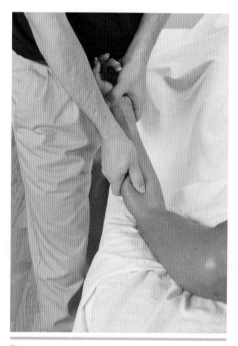

SEQUENCE 7-1 FIGURE 4

SUPINATOR

Apply compressive strokes and slow, deep stripping to the supinator. While compressing the supinator, rotate the wrist from supination to pronation.

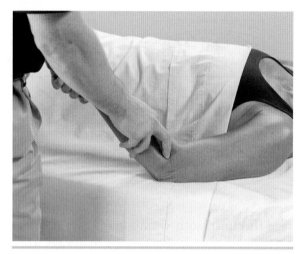

SEQUENCE 7-1 FIGURE 5

STRETCHING

Stretch the muscles of the arm and the wrists. Focus of the stretches should be on the flexors and extensors.

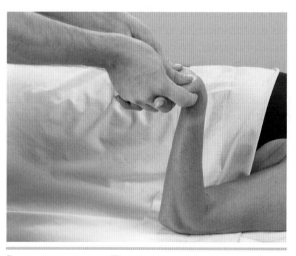

SEQUENCE 7-1 FIGURE 6

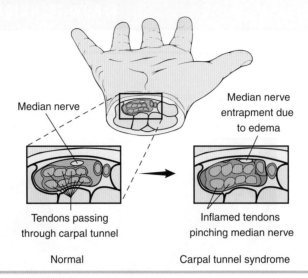

Median nerve

Median nerve entrapment due to edema

Tendons passing through carpal tunnel

Inflamed tendons pinching median nerve

Normal

Carpal tunnel syndrome

FIGURE 7-6 ■ Carpal tunnel syndrome. From Frazier MS, Drzymkowski JW: *Essentials of human diseases and conditions,* ed 2, Philadelphia, 2000, WB Saunders.)

average massage therapist, so it is important to refer the client to his or her doctor for an official diagnosis. Remember to always work within your scope of practice.

Although the carpal tunnel is located in the wrist, the tendons of the flexor group are most often affected. Working the flexor group from the wrist to the elbow is important. Similar to epicondylitis, fascial work, kneading, and trigger-point approaches to the flexors of the wrist aid in returning the muscles to their normal resting positions. Stripping the palmar surface along with broadening the carpal area can help stretch the flexor retinaculum, which can alleviate some of the pressure on the median nerve. **Distraction**, or **traction**, of the wrist can also be beneficial; however, be cautious of the force being used as you may dislocate the wrist. Slow, consistent pressure should be used in a linear motion. It is important to pull to the point of resistance and avoid twisting during this motion. Digital compression with active and passive motions to the flexor group and stretching of this group will aid in returning the muscles to their normal resting position (Sequence 7-2).

SEQUENCE 7-2

WARM UP

Use pétrissage to warm up the tissues of the arm and forearm. Use broadening strokes and deep slides from distal to proximal on the forearm to loosen the tissue.

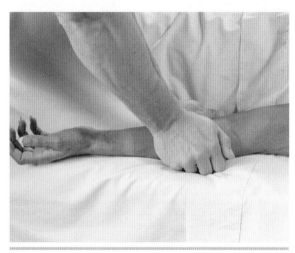

SEQUENCE 7-2 FIGURE 1

PRONATOR TERES

Apply deep longitudinal slides to the pronator teres. Compress the pronator teres and move the hand from pronation to supination.

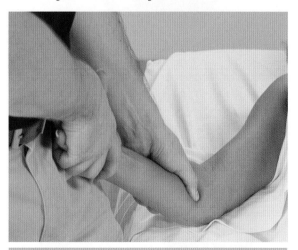

SEQUENCE 7-2 FIGURE 2

CARPAL TUNNEL SEQUENCE

FLEXOR AND EXTENSOR TENDONS

Apply deep, multidirectional friction to the common extensor and flexor tendons.

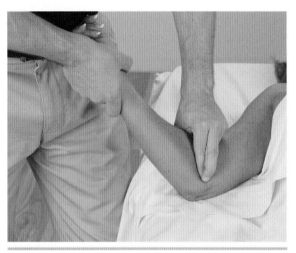

SEQUENCE 7-2 FIGURE 3

FLEXOR RETINACULUM

Apply longitudinal strokes moving from midline to lateral and multidirectional friction to the flexor retinaculum.

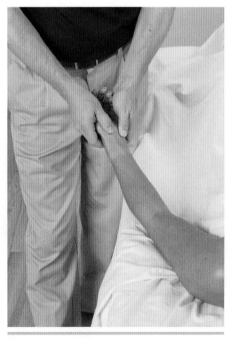

SEQUENCE 7-2 FIGURE 4

PALMAR APONEUROSIS

Interlace your fingers with the client's and apply broadening strokes to the palmar aponeurosis and friction between the metacarpals.

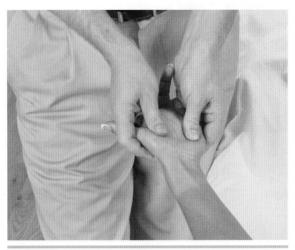

SEQUENCE 7-2 FIGURE 5

STRETCHING

Stretch the muscles of the wrist and hand by extending the wrist and flexing the elbow. Open the hand to enhance the stretch.

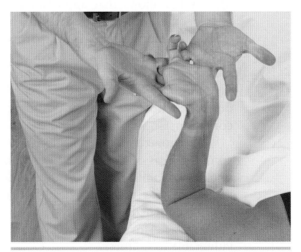

SEQUENCE 7-2 FIGURE 6

CHAPTER 8

BACK AND ABDOMINALS

OUTLINE

KEY TERMS

axial skeleton
Davis' law
deep layer
deepest layer
flattening of the spine
forward head
functional scoliosis
hyperkyphosis
hyperlordosis
hypertonicity
kyphosis
lordosis
lower crossed syndrome
muscular layers
pelvis
postural distortions
scoliosis
structural scoliosis
superficial layer
thoracopelvic region
thorax
upper crossed syndrome
Wolff's law

OBJECTIVES

1   Understand the anatomy of the thoracopelvic region.
2   Explain the muscular layers of the back.
3   Understand the natural curvatures of the spine.
4   Define the common postural distortions.
5   Understand the anatomy of the abdominal area.
6   Explain considerations about working with postural distortions.

Studies shows that approximately four out of five people will complain about back pain at some point during their life. Approximately 31 million Americans are experiencing back pain at any given moment. The causes of this pain are not usually due to direct insult or injury (acute trauma), but are more often due to repetitive stress, poor posture, or overuse (chronic conditions).

The thorax and pelvic regions are some of the more complex areas of the body. Whereas most muscles cross one or two joints, muscles of the **thorax** often cross multiple joints like the vertebrae. Multiarticulating muscles are not designed to be fully lengthened over all joints at one time. This limited extensibility makes them more vulnerable to injuries.

The thorax is heavily layered with muscles that serve not only to create specific actions, but also to maintain posture and balance and protect vital organs. Understanding this complex network of fascia, muscles, ligaments, and articulations is important in deep tissue massage approaches and techniques.

ANATOMY OF THE THORACOPELVIC REGION

Although this is not an anatomy text, it is important to review the anatomy of the **thoracopelvic region** to understand the complaints that clients express. The foundation of this area is composed of the vertebral spine, rib cage, **pelvis**, sacrum, and coccyx (Figure 8-1). It is structurally held together by a complex network of ligaments, fascia, tendons, and muscles. Multiple moving parts and the shape of this area make it more prone to injury, especially repetitive-movement disorders. Poor posture and incorrect body mechanics lead to trauma, repetitive injuries, stress disorders, and muscular pain.

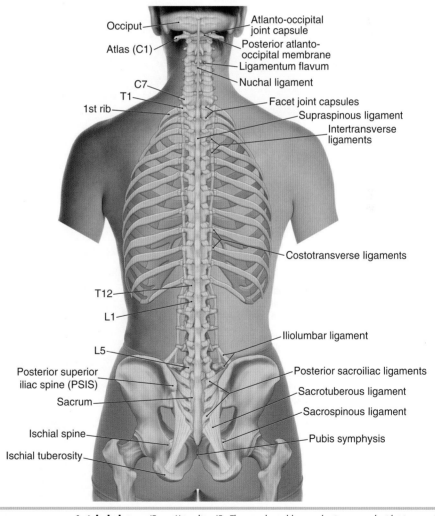

FIGURE 8-1 ■ **Axial skeleton.** (From Muscolino JE: *The muscle and bone palpation manual with trigger points, referral patterns, and stretching,* St Louis, 2009, Mosby.)

The musculature of the back can be classified into three levels of depth: **superficial**, **deep**, and **deepest**. This is a key understanding to successful deep tissue massage. Not all the smaller, intricate muscles of the thorax are listed because they are beyond the scope of this text; however, the focus of the massage therapist is on the following layers of muscles.

The deepest layer consists of the postural muscles, which many therapists strive to address. These consist of the suboccipitals, transversospinalis group (multifidi, rotators, and semispinalis), and intercostalis muscles (Figure 8-2).

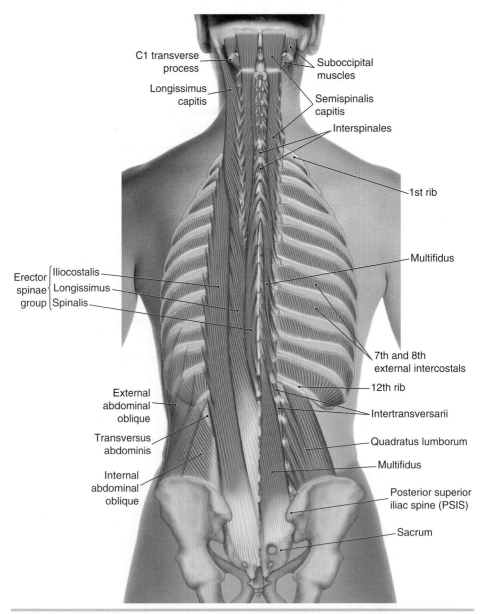

FIGURE 8-2 ■ Deepest layer. (From Muscolino JE: *The muscle and bone palpation manual with trigger points, referral patterns, and stretching,* St Louis, 2009, Mosby.)

The deep layer consists of the splenius (capitis, cervicis), levator scapulae, erector spinae group (iliocostalis, longissimus, spinalis), serratus posterior (superior and inferior). This is the area where most therapists spend their time working (Figure 8-3).

The superficial layer consists of the trapezius, rhomboids, latissimus dorsi, and serratus anterior (Figure 8-4).

Visualizing the back of the body in context to the **muscular layers** helps the therapist understand the three-dimensional complex of the body. Identifying which muscles need to be addressed dictates the appropriate layer to focus on. The layer being addressed dictates the depth, pressure, and speed of the technique. Understanding this process helps identify the approach and technique that is best suited for the muscle.

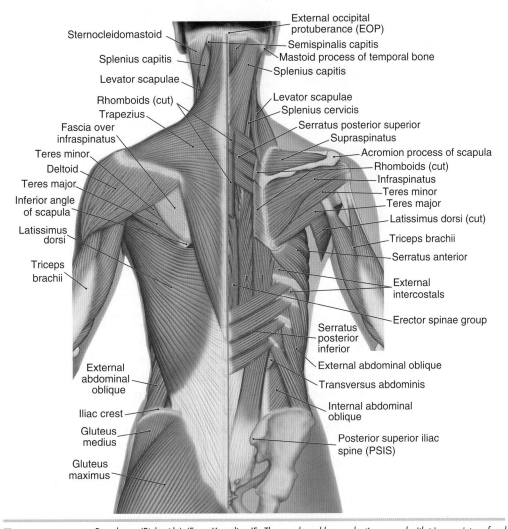

FIGURE 8-3 ■ Deep layer. (Right side) (From Muscolino JE: *The muscle and bone palpation manual with trigger points, referral patterns, and stretching,* St Louis, 2009, Mosby.)

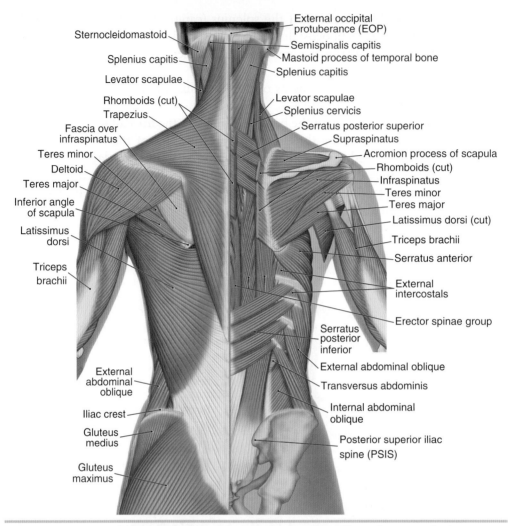

FIGURE 8-4 ■ Superficial layer. (Left side) (From Muscolino JE: *The muscle and bone palpation manual with trigger points, referral patterns, and stretching,* St Louis, 2009, Mosby.)

POSTURAL DISTORTIONS

Some of the causes of back discomfort can be directly related to **postural distortions** of some form. Postural distortions were discussed briefly in Chapter 2 about the assessment of the client. As discussed, hyperlordosis, hyperkyphosis, and scoliosis are distortions of concern. However, that chapter did not discuss how those distortions are created. Many therapists have been trained to think of these misalignments in the form of a linear positioning of the spine.

In hyperkyphosis, for example, the outward curvature is increased, creating a rounded back. This happens only in the thoracic area. The majority of spinal curvatures are due to rotations in the vertebrae, which result in an additional or accentuated curve. These rotations can happen anywhere in the spine; *lordosis, kyphosis,* and *scoliosis* refer only to the direction of the curvature.

Understanding the effects of daily activities on the body is also important. The question becomes one of structure and function. According to **Wolff's law and Davis' Law**, changes in the function of the body are followed by changes in the structure. During the assessment and health history, one should explore the underlying issue, and whether the pain is due to structural abnormalities or whether it is due to poor posture (Box 8-1).

Postural distortions may be caused by birth defects, bone development, or habitual patterns created over time. It is important to understand that there is no "quick fix" when it comes to working on body alignment (Figure 8-5).

KYPHOTIC CURVES

The term **kyphosis** refers to any outward curvature of the spine. The thoracic region has a natural kyphotic curve ranging between 20 to 40 degrees. In **hyperkyphosis** the curvature exceeds 40 degrees. Some clients may present themselves with a cervical kyphosis, or hypolordosis. This is more commonly known as a straightening of the neck or **forward head** position. Some people have also used the terms *reverse angle* or *reverse curvature* to describe this disorder; however, these terms are not an accurate description. The lumbar area can also become kyphotic, or hypolordotic; this is known as a *flat back*.

Box 8-1   WOLFF'S LAW AND DAVIS' LAW OF BONE ADAPTATION

Wolff's law describes the principle that every change in the form and function of a bone or in the function of the bone alone leads to changes in its internal architecture and in its external form.

Wolff's law states that skeletal transformation depends on the exertion of pressures from outside sources. Whereas Davis' law explains how soft tissues remodel themselves according to the demands put on them from outside sources.

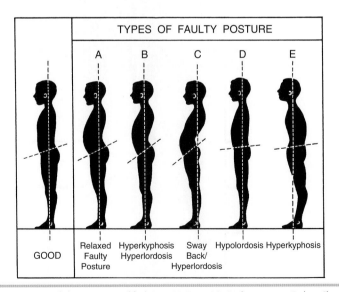

FIGURE 8-5 ■ Postural distortions. (Modified From McMorris RO: Faulty postures, *Pediatr Clin North Am* 8:217, 1961.)

Although hyperkyphosis may be caused by congenital defects, it is more commonly a result of developmental or progressive disorders. It is often the result of degenerative disk disorders, habitual postural deviations, or osteoporosis, to name a few possibilities. Hyperkyphosis may present several different postural deviations that are of concern. A forward head posture is commonly seen with hyperkyphosis. This position increases the muscular tension in the posterior neck muscles and may increase the lordotic curvature of the cervical spine. This curvature can also cause a compression of the ribcage, which can affect the functions of the respiratory and digestive systems and increase tension in the upper chest muscles (Figure 8-6) (Sequence 8-1).

LORDOTIC CURVES

Lordosis is a term used to describe the inward curves in the spine commonly found in the lumbar and cervical areas. The cervical area has a lordotic range of 20-35 degrees and the lumbar ranges between 40-60 degrees. When the curvature exceeds these ranges it is considered **hyperlordosis**. If the curvature is less than these ranges, therapists use the terms *straightening* or **flattening of the spine**. Normal aging process, poor posture, or developmental or progressive disorders may result in a straightening of these curves, or hyperlordosis (Sequence 8-2).

Poor posture and activities of daily living are major contributors of hyperlordosis. Hyperlordosis of the lumbar region can be due to the shortening or tight hip flexors. This is common in people who sit at a desk for the majority of the day. In the seated position the psoas and iliacus muscles are in a shortened state. They become trained to be this length, and fascia can become restricted.

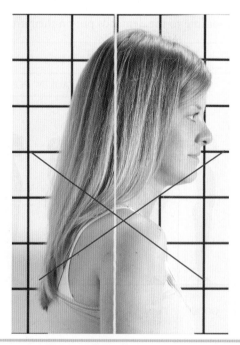

FIGURE 8-6 ■ Tight muscles of hyperkyphosis. Weak: deep neck flexors, rhomboids, and serratus anterior. Shortened: pectoralis, trapezius, and levator scapula.

Text continued on p. 130

SEQUENCE 8-1

WARM UP TISSUES OF THE UPPER TORSO

Warm up the tissues of the anterior chest using effleurage and myofascial stretching.

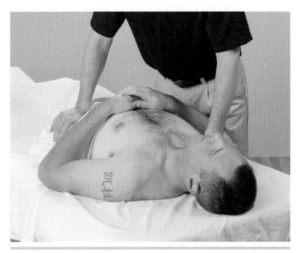

SEQUENCE 8-1 FIGURE 1

PECTORALIS MAJOR

Address the needs of the pectoralis muscles. Kneading and deep glides from medial to lateral aid in lengthening these shortened muscles. Transverse friction at the insertion also benefits the elongation of this muscle.

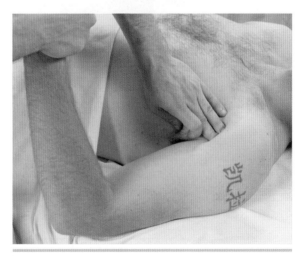

SEQUENCE 8-1 FIGURE 2

PECTORALIS MINOR

The pectoralis minor is often overlooked in regard to its role in **upper crossed syndrome**. Slow slides and compression are good techniques to use.

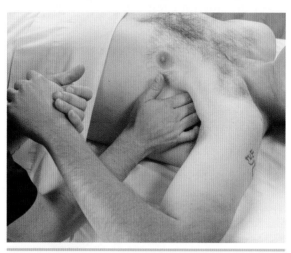

SEQUENCE 8-1 FIGURE 3

LATISSIMUS DORSI

Lengthening the latissimus dorsi is also beneficial. Transverse friction at its insertion will also help relax the muscle.

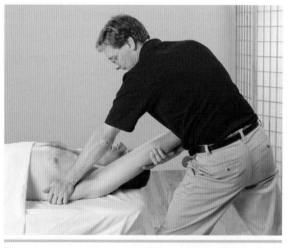

SEQUENCE 8-1 FIGURE 4

LEVATOR SCAPULAE

Kneading and stripping strokes from superior to inferior along with transverse friction at the insertions of this muscle helps relax this muscle. Stretching is also beneficial for the levators.

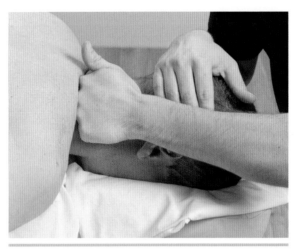

SEQUENCE 8–1 FIGURE 5

TRAPEZIUS

Knead and strip the upper trapezius muscles. Deep stripping strokes from origin to insertion and transverse friction also aid in elongation of this muscle.

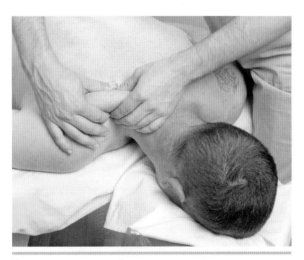

SEQUENCE 8–1 FIGURE 6

HYPERKYPHOSIS SEQUENCE

RHOMBOIDS AND SERRATUS

It is important to stimulate the rhomboids and reposition the shoulder into its natural position. This can be done by lifting the shoulder or propping the shoulder with a towel. Then address the needs of the rhomboids with a more stimulating technique.

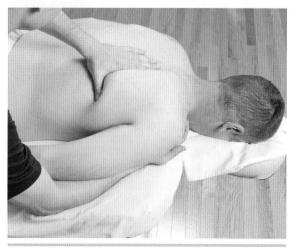

SEQUENCE 8-1 FIGURE 7

STRETCHING AND CIRCULATION

End the sequence with effleurage to encourage circulation, and with stretching. The stretching should focus on opening the chest cavity.

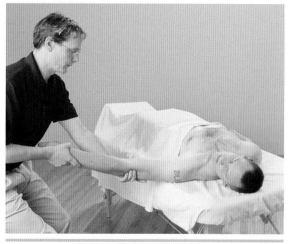

SEQUENCE 8-1 FIGURE 8

SEQUENCE 8-2

WARM UP

Warm up the tissues of the lower back with effleurage, pétrissage, and myofascial techniques.

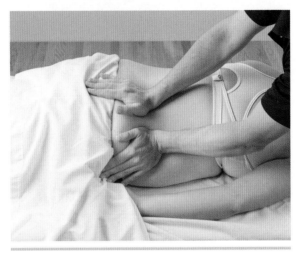

SEQUENCE 8-2 FIGURE 1

ERECTOR SPINAE

Use rocking compression, stripping strokes, and friction to remove restrictions in the thoracolumbar fascia and erectors, focusing on the longissimus muscles.

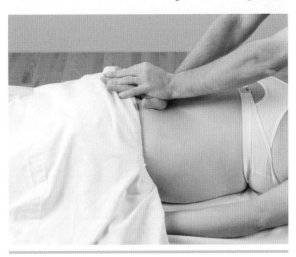

SEQUENCE 8-2 FIGURE 2

HYPERLORDOSIS SEQUENCE

QUADRATUS LUMBORUM

Apply broadening strokes and stripping strokes to the quadratus lumborum. Friction and transverse strokes along the iliac crest are also effective techniques.

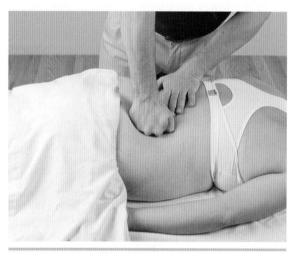

SEQUENCE 8-2 FIGURE 3

PSOAS

Access the psoas in the supine or side-lying position. Use active movements to engage the psoas to help relax the muscle.

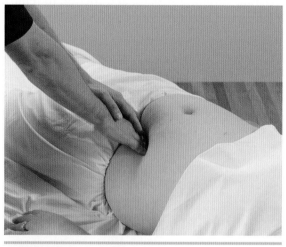

SEQUENCE 8-2 FIGURE 4

GLUTEAL MUSCLES

Apply pétrissage and stimulating techniques to the gluteal muscles. Use active and passive movements with compression to release restrictions in the muscles.

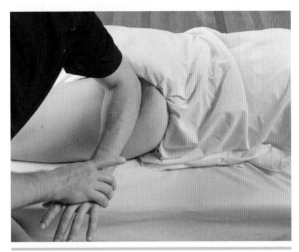

SEQUENCE 8-2 FIGURE 5

STRETCHING

End the sequence with stretching of the psoas and low back muscles.

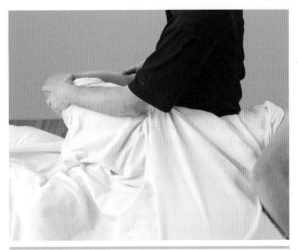

SEQUENCE 8-2 FIGURE 6

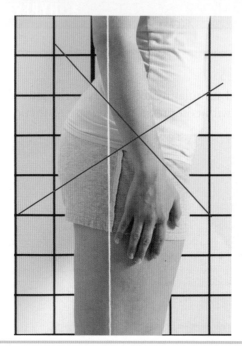

FIGURE 8-7 ■ Tight muscles of hyperlordosis. Weak: gluteus maximus and abdominals. Shortened: erector spinae and iliopsoas groups.

When the person stands, the muscles do not want to stretch, which could pull the anterior surface of the lumbar vertebrae forward, increasing the lordotic curve (Figure 8-7).

SCOLIOSIS

Scoliosis is a general term referring to lateral curvatures in the spine. A more appropriate description of scoliosis is a condition involving a rotation of the spinal column resulting in a distinctive lateral curvature (Figure 8-8). This condition is relatively common with children and is often due to muscular imbalances or disease. In **structural scoliosis** there are actual deformities in the vertebrae. This is a genetic disorder and usually requires surgical intervention such as rods.

Functional scoliosis is a result of muscular imbalances such as **hypertonicity** of the quadratus lumborum, erector spinae, and transversospinalis muscle groups. Although muscular tension is a leading cause of functional scoliosis, minor structural abnormalities may also contribute to the imbalances like leg lengths. Assessment of the client's skeletal system prior to muscular assessment is important to plan an effective treatment plan.

LOW BACK PAIN

As stated earlier, there are approximately 31 million people experiencing back pain at any given moment. The causes of low back pain can be as diverse as the people experiencing the pain. Muscular tightness, overstretching, ligament

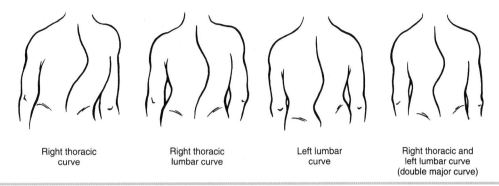

Right thoracic
curve

Right thoracic
lumbar curve

Left lumbar
curve

Right thoracic and
left lumbar curve
(double major curve)

FIGURE 8-8 ▦ Scoliotic curvatures. (From Barkauskas VH et al: *Health and physical assessment,* ed 3, St Louis, 2002, Mosby.)

or tendon trauma, inflammation, structural deviations, postural patterns, and disease and disorders may cause generalized pain and discomfort. A clear understanding of the pain the client is experiencing along with a thorough assessment is essential to understanding the source of the pain.

As this pain is such a broad subject, this section focuses on the common muscular changes experienced with low back pain. Dr. Vladimir Janda popularized what is referred to as the **lower crossed syndrome**. This term describes the predictable muscular changes caused by a shift in pelvic positioning. A client with lower crossed syndrome, which is mostly associated with an anterior tilt in the pelvis, shows signs of shortening in the quadratus lumborum, longissimus, iliopsoas, and rectus femoris. Dr. Janda stated that because of reciprocal inhibition the antagonist of the short muscle will lengthen, creating weakness. These weak muscles are the rectus abdominis and core muscles and the gluteal muscle group. This change in the pelvis angle, hyperlordosis, and muscular imbalance make the individual more susceptible to future injuries that are likely to be more severe.

ABDOMINALS

It is said that the secret to a strong back is strong abdominals. This phrase and society's impression of a flat, "six-pack" abdominal region as the desired look has sent many people to the gym to dedicate a portion of their workouts to abdominal crunches. Thankfully health and fitness trainers are supporting the focus of abdominal strengthening toward the "core" group, including the obliques and the transversus abdominis. Even when the focus of abdominal work is on stabilization, too much work on these muscles can lead to an imbalance of the trunk and cause postural deviations.

Working superficially to deep, these muscles are the rectus abdominis, which runs from the ribcage to the pubic symphysis. The internal and external obliques run along the sides of the trunk at angles and the transversus abdominis is the deepest layer, running perpendicular to the rectus abdominis (Figure 8-9). The transversus abdominis is the body's natural back brace.

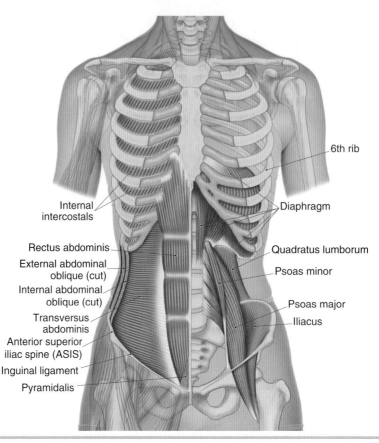

FIGURE 8-9 ▪ Abdominal muscles. (From Muscolino JE: *The muscle and bone palpation manual with trigger points, referral patterns, and stretching,* St Louis, 2009, Mosby.)

Understanding the direction of these fibers is important when working these layers. To help visualize how these core muscles protect the organs and abdominal cavity, it also helps to understand how important these muscles work in core stability and balance.

WORKING WITH POSTURE

When working on the back, one of the key thoughts to keep in mind is to return the body to balance. Although one can get distracted working the tight muscles and trigger points, remember that it is only part of the equation. For every tight muscle you find, there is also a muscle locked in an elongated position. For example, before spending a lot of time working on the trapezius because of tension and soreness, do not neglect stretching and releasing the pectoral muscles first. We are effective in returning the trapezius to its normal resting position only if the pectoral allows the shoulders to realign.

When working a lateral curvature, the concave portion of the curve appears tight and hypertonic whereas the convex portion is weak and long. It is important to bring balance to this agonist-antagonist relationship. The choice of technique used and direction of the stroke play important roles. Always be aware of any contraindications or limitations the client may have, especially when addressing spinal curvatures. Clients who are older than the age of 20 may have structural abnormalities; the client may also exhibit hypersensitivity, which will prevent a deep approach to care. Although treatment of true scoliosis may show limited results, a slight lateral curvature caused by different leg lengths can be compensated for to aid in reducing low back pain.

CHAPTER 9

HIPS AND THIGHS

OBJECTIVES

1   Describe the musculoskeletal design of the pelvic girdle.
2   Define and identify the muscles of the hip.
3   Demonstrate techniques for the psoas muscle.
4   Explain and identify common disorders of the hips and thighs.

The **pelvis**, a crucial region of the body, is the area where the lower extremities attach to the axial skeleton through the sacroiliac (SI) joint. The pelvis houses parts of the digestive system and the urinary and reproductive systems. The lower extremities, the trunk, and the spinal column can influence the movements and position of the pelvis, and the positioning of the pelvis can influence the movements and positioning of the lower extremities, the trunk, and the spinal column. Deep **postural muscles** in this area work hard to maintain spinal **stability** and proper positioning. This region also contains muscles that can be difficult to access because of the depth at which they are located. Tightness in these muscles can pull the body out of its ideal position. For example, tightness in the gluteal or deep lateral rotator muscles can cause the hip to laterally rotate. This lateral rotation commonly results in a shift of the sacrum, which hikes the hip on the affected side. If there is tightness bilaterally, this may result in a posterior pelvic tilt, which can lead to a flat back or a decrease in the lordotic curvature of the lumbar vertebrae. This flat back syndrome may be a precursor to **hyperkyphosis** of the thoracic area.

Because of this tension in the gluteal and "deep six" musculature, clients may experience low back pain and possibly even headaches.

MUSCLES OF THE HIP AND THIGH

GLUTEAL GROUP

On the posterior aspect of the pelvis are the gluteal muscles. Working superficial to deep and posterior to lateral, there are three gluteal muscles: gluteus maximus, gluteus medius, and the gluteus minimus. These muscles help stabilize the upper body, aid in locomotion, and extend the hip. Originating from the sacrum, the gluteus maximus is a key muscle that ties the leg to the pelvis (Figure 9-1).

Although the **iliotibial (IT) band or tract** runs the length of the lateral thigh, we are including it as part of the hip because it acts as one of the insertion points of the gluteus maximus. The IT band also acts as an attachment site for the **tensor fascia latae (TFL)**. The TFL is a hip abductor and has an important role as a hip stabilizer (Figure 9-2).

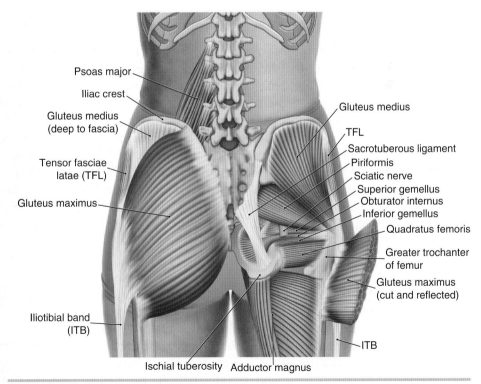

FIGURE 9-1 ■ Gluteal muscles. (From Muscolino JE: *The muscle and bone palpation manual with trigger points, referral patterns, and stretching,* St Louis, 2009, Mosby.)

135

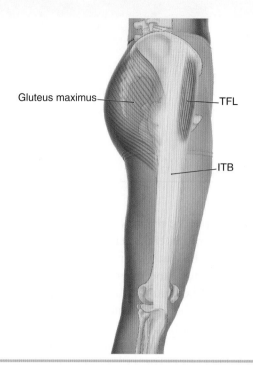

Gluteus maximus

TFL

ITB

FIGURE 9-2 ■ Tensor fascia latae and iliotibial band. (From Muscolino JE: *The muscle and bone palpation manual with trigger points, referral patterns, and stretching,* St Louis, 2009, Mosby.)

DEEP LATERAL ROTATORS

The **deep lateral rotators**, often referred to as the **deep six muscles**, are a group of six muscles that lie under the gluteal group. These muscles play an important role in stabilizing the pelvis and rotation of the hip. These muscles are the piriformis, gemellus superior, obturator internus, gemellus inferior, obturator externus, and quadratus femoris. This small group of muscles is a major culprit in low back and leg pain. The piriformis muscle originates from the anterior surface of the sacrum and attaches to the greater trochanter of the femur. It uses the femur as a counterbalance to maintain spinal positioning through the sacrum. Because of its positioning, the tendency to become tight and compress the sciatic nerve is common. The quadratus femoris originates from the ischial tuberosity and is often tight and tender to touch when worked (Figure 9-3).

HIP FLEXORS

The hip flexors help balance the posterior pelvic muscles. Three key muscles often become tight and shortened as a result of activities of daily living. These are the iliacus, psoas major, and the rectus femoris. The iliacus and the psoas major are often referred to as the *iliopsoas* because they share the same insertion at the lesser trochanter of the femur. The psoas minor inserts on the superior ramus of the pubis bone and mainly supports the natural lordotic curvature of the spine, but is only found in about 40% of the population. The psoas major originates on the anterior surface of the lumbar vertebrae and runs over

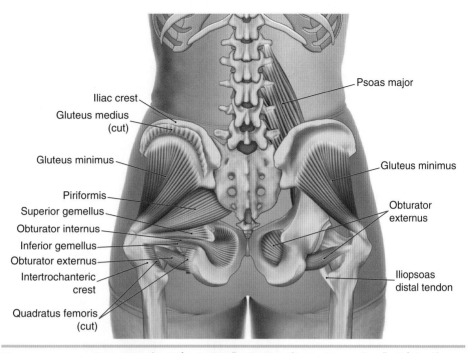

FIGURE 9-3 ■ Deep six muscles: Piriformis, Gemellus Superior, Obturator Internus, Gemellus Inferior, Obturator Externus, and Quadratus Femoris. (From Muscolino JE: *The muscle and bone palpation manual with trigger points, referral patterns, and stretching,* St Louis, 2009, Mosby.)

the pubis bone and inserts into the lesser trochanter of the femur. This muscle not only helps to flex the hip, but also has an effect on the lordotic curvature of the lumbar vertebrae. The rectus femoris has a proximal attachment at the **acetabulum** and inserts into the tibial tuberosity. This long muscle plays a role in both hip flexion and leg extension (Figure 9-4).

When these muscles are under constant tension because of **ergonomics** and habitual **postural positioning**, they may become tight and shortened. This can result in pulling forward on the lumbar vertebrae, creating **hyperlordosis** and causing the pelvis to tilt anteriorly. This is commonly seen in people who maintain a seated position for a prolonged period such as office workers, computer programmers, and others who find themselves sitting at a desk for hours every day. It is important to provide education on proper ergonomics, movement, and self-care to these individuals.

Working in the pelvic region is not easy for many therapists and clients. There are cautions and **borders** that need to be addressed and talked through before addressing these muscles. There are emotional and comfort aspects about working in the lower pelvic region. Some clients find this area too personal or private to allow the therapist's hands in this area. Other considerations are the internal organs such as the intestines, uterus, kidneys, and bladder. As the iliacus and psoas travel under the inguinal ligament and insert into the lesser trochanter of the femur, there is also the femoral triangle, which needs to be worked around. Body positioning can be useful to help access these muscles in a less invasive way while protecting the comfort of the client.

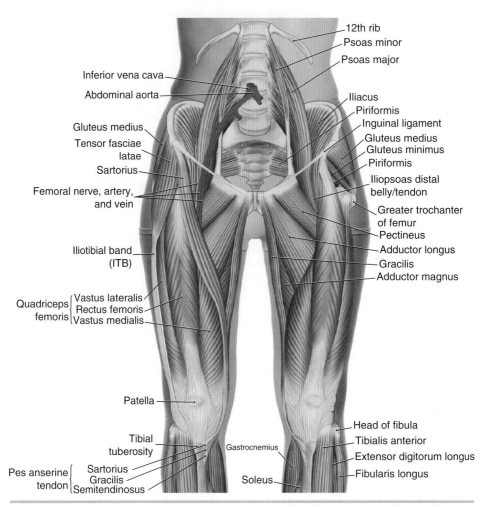

FIGURE 9-4 ■ Hip flexors. (From Muscolino JE: *The muscle and bone palpation manual with trigger points, referral patterns, and stretching,* St Louis, 2009, Mosby.)

MUSCLES OF THE THIGH

For the purposes of this text, when referring to the thigh we are referring to the musculature of the upper portion of the leg, between the hip and the knee. These muscles play important roles in the leg and hip positioning. Leg position and leg lengths can have a dramatic effect on the pelvic alignment, which affects the spinal alignment. An internally or externally rotated hip can have an effect not only on the pelvic position, but also on the client's gait. A thorough assessment helps determine which muscles are tight or restricted; working from the feet up to the pelvis may help determine the focus of the session (Figure 9-5).

QUADRICEPS

The quadriceps group consists of four muscles: rectus femoris, vastus lateralis, vastus medialis, and vastus intermedius. All four muscles work together to perform knee extension; however, the rectus femoris also plays a role in hip flexion. The rectus femoris is a biarticulate muscle, meaning it passes over two

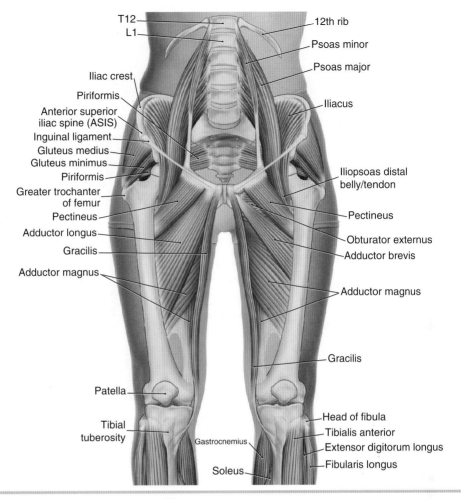

T12
L1
Iliac crest
Piriformis
Anterior superior
iliac spine (ASIS)
Inguinal ligament
Gluteus medius
Gluteus minimus
Piriformis
Greater trochanter
of femur
Pectineus
Adductor longus
Gracilis
Adductor magnus
Patella
Tibial
tuberosity

12th rib
Psoas minor
Psoas major
Iliacus
Iliopsoas distal
belly/tendon
Pectineus
Obturator externus
Adductor brevis
Adductor magnus
Gracilis
Head of fibula
Tibialis anterior
Extensor digitorum longus
Fibularis longus
Gastrocnemius
Soleus

FIGURE 9-4 ▦ cont'd.

joints: the knee and hip. Its main function is as a knee extender; however, the proximal attachment at the anterior inferior iliac spine and the acetabulum allows for this muscle to act as a hip flexor as well. Distally, all four muscles merge together to form the quadriceps tendon. This tendon continues to its attachment point at the tibial tuberosity. The patella is engulfed in this tendon and aids in allowing the tendon to track properly during movement (Figure 9-6).

HAMSTRINGS

The hamstrings are a group of three muscles on the posterior aspect of the leg. All three muscles attach proximally at the ischial tuberosity of the pelvis. The bicep femoris inserts distally into the lateral epicondyle of the tibia. The semitendinosus and the semimembranosus share the same insertion onto the medial aspect of the tibia through the pes anserinus tendon. The hamstrings serve two main actions: knee flexion and hip extension (Figure 9-7). Hamstrings that are tight and short pull on the ischial tuberosity when standing, which can result in drawing the pelvis down, rotating it posteriorly. This posterior rotation can encourage a flattening of the lumbar curvature, which may lead to hyperkyphosis and a forward head.

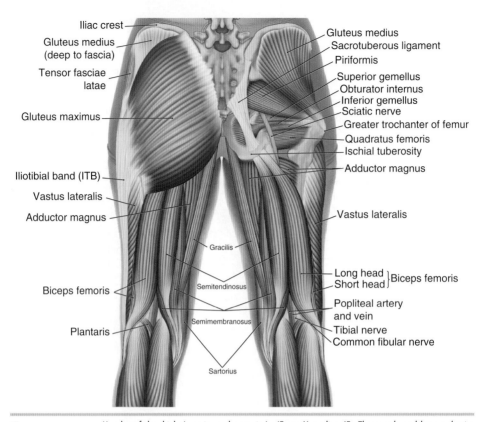

FIGURE 9-5 ■ Muscles of the thigh (anterior and posterior). (From Muscolino JE: *The muscle and bone palpation manual with trigger points, referral patterns, and stretching,* St Louis, 2009, Mosby.)

ADDUCTORS

The *adductor muscles* refer to five muscles: pectineus, gracilis, adductor longus, adductor brevis, and adductor magnus. In addition, the sartorius is responsible for multiple actions at the hip and knee, including assisting in adduction of the hip. Although these muscles are associated with their main actions, which is adduction of the hip, the adductor magnus also plays a key role in stabilizing the knee when the hamstrings are engaged. If the hamstrings are weak or restricted, the adductors will kick in to help with the actions and movement of the knee (Figure 9-8).

BALANCING THE HIP

As discussed briefly in Chapter 2, **lower crossed syndrome** causes the hip flexors and the low back muscles to become tight, short, and restricted, and their antagonist muscles to become long and weak. This results in the pelvis tilting anteriorly, creating a hyperlordotic posture. Many therapists attempt to address this postural shift by working the quadratus lumborum and lower aspects of the erector spinae group. This, however, is only a portion of the equation. If we do not address the hip flexors with more than stretching they will pull the pelvis back into this anterior tilted position.

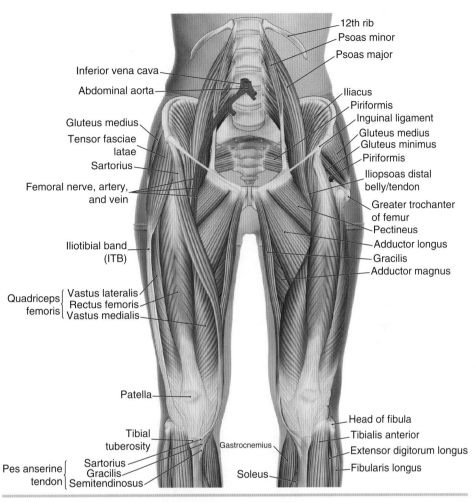

12th rib
Psoas minor
Psoas major
Inferior vena cava
Abdominal aorta
Iliacus
Piriformis
Inguinal ligament
Gluteus medius
Tensor fasciae latae
Gluteus medius
Gluteus minimus
Piriformis
Sartorius
Iliopsoas distal belly/tendon
Femoral nerve, artery, and vein
Greater trochanter of femur
Pectineus
Adductor longus
Gracilis
Adductor magnus
Iliotibial band (ITB)
Quadriceps femoris { Vastus lateralis / Rectus femoris / Vastus medialis }
Patella
Head of fibula
Tibial tuberosity
Tibialis anterior
Extensor digitorum longus
Gastrocnemius
Fibularis longus
Pes anserine tendon { Sartorius / Gracilis / Semitendinosus }
Soleus

FIGURE 9-5 ▥ cont'd.

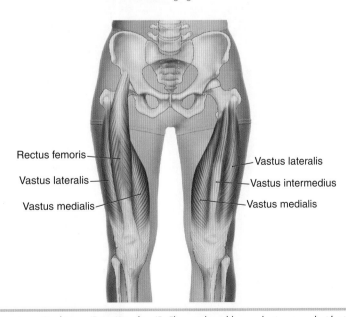

Rectus femoris
Vastus lateralis
Vastus lateralis
Vastus intermedius
Vastus medialis
Vastus medialis

FIGURE 9-6 ▥ Quadriceps. (From Muscolino JE: *The muscle and bone palpation manual with trigger points, referral patterns, and stretching,* St Louis, 2009, Mosby.)

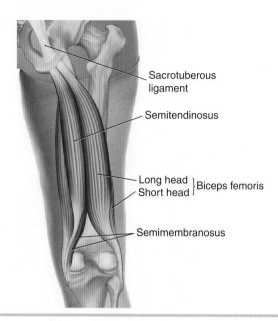

FIGURE 9-7 ■ Hamstrings. (From Muscolino JE: *The muscle and bone palpation manual with trigger points, referral patterns, and stretching,* St Louis, 2009, Mosby.)

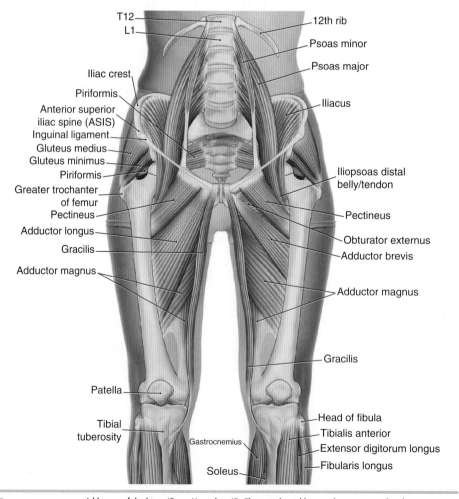

FIGURE 9-8 ■ Adductors of the hips. (From Muscolino JE: *The muscle and bone palpation manual with trigger points, referral patterns, and stretching,* St Louis, 2009, Mosby.)

PSOAS

As with any deep tissue technique, the deeper you enter the body, the slower the technique becomes. Accessing the psoas muscle from a side-lying position allows the therapist to release and stretch the muscle without having to change the client's position. Gravity helps by shifting the organs down and out of the way of the access point. The psoas is a deep muscle and cannot be manipulated like superficial muscles using techniques like effleurage; compression becomes the most effective technique to use. Adding active and passive range of motion helps to release this muscle.

The entry point for the therapist is approximately 1 inch medial to the anterior superior iliac spine. The direction of the pressure is inward toward the anterior aspect of the lumbar vertebrae. Passively move the hip into flexion to aid in softening the skin and musculature of the hip flexors. If you are unsure if you are on the psoas muscle, have the client contract it by flexing the hip against your resistance. Make any adjustments necessary and hold that compression. Passively move the hip from flexion to extension with this compression. Repeat as necessary while relocating your fingers along the psoas muscle. Finish with stretching the psoas by supporting the low back with your hip and moving the hip into extension.

Another approach is with the client supine. Starting approximately 1 inch medial to the anterior superior iliac spine, apply a downward pressure toward the anterior surface of the lumbar vertebrae. Caution needs to be exercised here because of the pelvic organs, especially the ovaries in females. Have the client bend the knee to help soften the skin and fascia of the lower pelvic area. This will help to get your fingers to the correct depth. This position does not allow for extension of the hip; however, it is more conducive for active movements. While compressing the tissues, have the client execute a straight leg raise approximately 9 inches to 1 foot off the table. The client should then relax as you passively return the leg to the table. After approximately three leg raises, rather than slowly returning the leg to the table, let the leg drop to the table. This helps engage more proprioceptors of the hip (Sequence 9-1).

After releasing and lengthening the psoas, the next muscles to address are the low back muscles, especially the quadratus lumborum and the lower erector spinae (see Chapter 8). Have the client walk around the room after techniques like this to become aware of the freedom of movement in the hips. The client must be aware of hip positioning as he or she moves to help reprogram these muscles.

QUADRICEPS

The rectus femoris not only acts on the pelvis as a hip flexor, but it also has a major role on the knee as a knee extender. Its attachment point on the anterior inferior iliac spine acts as a hip flexor, whereas its other proximal attachment at the acetabulum helps to anchor the femur to the pelvis. This has two effects on the pelvis: a pull on the pelvis to create an anterior tilt and compression of the hip at the joint. Because of these two effects, it is important to lengthen this muscle and free it of restrictions when it is tight.

According to basic massage training, strokes used should always encourage venous return and be administered toward the heart. Decompressing the hip is an example in which the intention of the stroke conflicts with basic teachings.

Text continued on p. 148

PSOAS RELEASE SEQUENCE

SEQUENCE 9-1

SUPINE POSITION

Warm Up

Use pétrissage to warm up the tissues of the hip and thigh. Perform a basic abdominal massage in a clockwise direction to help relax the abdominal cavity.

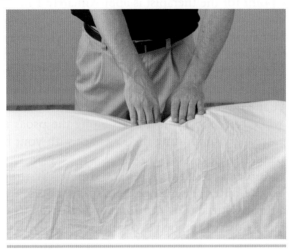

SEQUENCE 9–1 FIGURE 1

ACCESS THE PSOAS MAJOR

Place fingers approximately 0.5 inch to 1 inch medial to the anterior superior iliac spine. Apply digital pressure at downward and medial and slightly superior. Flex the hip by placing the client's foot flat on the table to help loosen the abdominopelvic area.

CAUTION

Move slowly; do not force the techniques. Be cautious of internal organs.

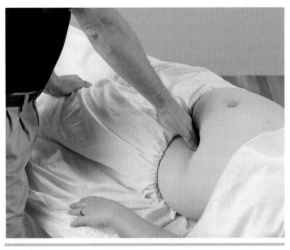

SEQUENCE 9–1 FIGURE 2

ACTIVE AND PASSIVE MOVEMENTS

Have the client flex the hip to activate the psoas muscle. This helps verify that you are on the psoas muscle. Have the client actively extend the hip and flex the hip. Apply slow longitudinal and transverse friction. With the leg extended, passively lift the leg approximately 6-9 inches and let it fall to the table. Do this three to five times.

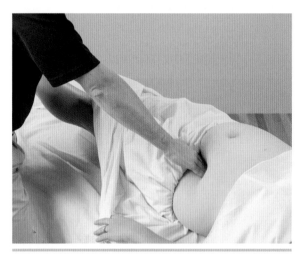

SEQUENCE 9-1 FIGURE 3

STRETCHING

Stretch the psoas and hip flexors, in the prone position. Use one hand or the forearm to stabilize the pelvis. Flex the knee and hold on to the thigh just above the knee. Extend the hip to the point of resistance.

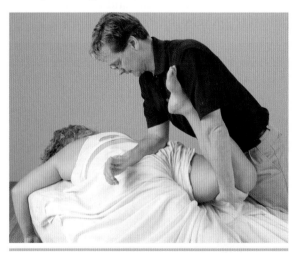

SEQUENCE 9-1 FIGURE 4

PSOAS RELEASE SEQUENCE

SIDE-LYING POSITION

Find The Landmarks

Place fingers approximately 0.5 inch to 1 inch medial to the anterior superior iliac spine. Apply digital pressure at downward and medial and slightly superior. Flex the hip to help loosen the abdominopelvic area.

CAUTION

Move slowly with this; do not force the techniques. Be cautious of internal organs.

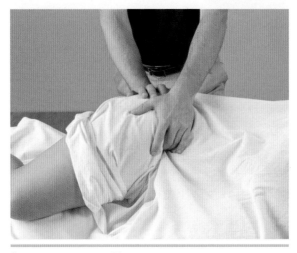

SEQUENCE 9-1 FIGURE 5

FRICTION AND COMPRESSION

With the hip flexed, apply slow longitudinal and transverse friction. Prop the hip with your arm or pillows to prevent the hips from moving.

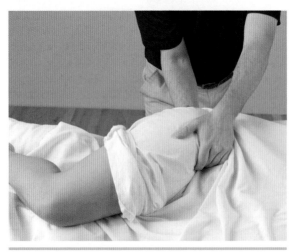

SEQUENCE 9-1 FIGURE 6

STRETCHING

Support the pelvic position by sitting with hip against sacrum. Hold on to the thigh just above the knee and the ankle. Extend the hip to elongate the psoas muscle. Flexing the knee during this motion will help to stretch all the hip flexors.

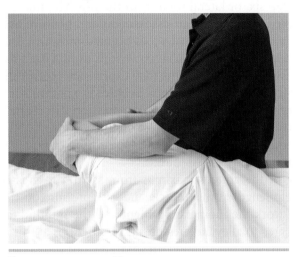

SEQUENCE 9-1 FIGURE 7

To decompress the hip joint, deep stripping strokes should be applied in a direction away from the hip. After working the quadriceps, lighter Swedish strokes like effleurage should be applied toward the heart to encourage venous flow. This is also a good application to transition to the next body part (Sequence 9-2).

DEEP SIX

There are two distinct visible characteristics when there is tightness and restriction in the deep six, or lateral rotators of the hip. The first and more prominent can be observed during the **gait assessment** and **posture assessment** when the client exhibits the duck walk with toes pointed outward. The second characteristic is a posterior pelvic tilt, which is obvious during the postural assessment.

Another symptom that clients may experience specifically with a shortened and tight piriformis muscle is sciatica. **Sciatica** is a pathologic condition in which the sciatic nerve is compressed. This compression can create numbness and tingling sensations down the posterior leg and may continue all the way to the feet. This impingement is often caused by the piriformis compressing the nerve or the nerve being pinched by the SI joint.

Stripping of the gluteus maximus from sacrum to greater trochanter of the femur can help lengthen this muscle and ease pressure on the SI joint. It is also important to work the iliosacral ligament and the multifidi and **thoracolumbar fascia** in this area to alleviate pressure and restrictions at this joint. Applying trigger point therapy and lengthening strokes to the piriformis can also help lessen the pressure on the sciatic nerve. Holding the trigger points while passively rotating the hip externally helps stretch and realign the piriformis muscle (Sequence 9-3).

KNEE JOINT

The knee joint is a complex hinge joint that is prone to injury because of its design. There are too many injuries and pathologic conditions of the knee to discuss fully in this book. We take a look at some common pathologic conditions that may come across the therapist's table.

Patellofemoral dysfunction results from an injury to the articulating surface between the patella and the femur. Discomfort from this disorder is often due to increased pressure and friction between the patella and the femur. If the patella does not track properly in the groove it can create friction on one side of the femur, creating pain and discomfort. This friction is often a result of restricted quadriceps muscles (Sequence 9-4).

Quadriceps dysfunction is a common term used for a variety of conditions that cause weakness, numbness, and cramping in the quadriceps muscles. Other signs may include reduced range of motion at the knee joint and knee pain. This disorder is often the result of trauma, overuse, strains, and may even be caused by inactivity.

Iliotibial band disorder is an inflammatory condition resulting from friction between the IT band and the femur. Although this disorder may be caused by a direct injury to the knee, it is most often caused by long-term overuse and friction. Symptoms of IT band disorder include aching and burning sensations in the lateral thigh and knee. Pain may radiate from the lateral hip down to the knee. Some people have mentioned that they feel or hear a "snap" at the knee when they extend the knee (Sequence 9-5).

QUADRICEPS SEQUENCE

SEQUENCE 9-2

WARM UP TISSUES

Use effleurage, pétrissage, and broadening strokes to warm the tissues of the thigh.

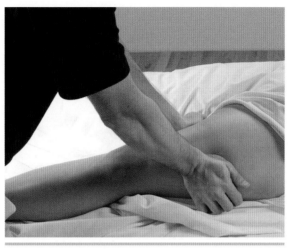

SEQUENCE 9-2 FIGURE 1

DECOMPRESSION OF THE HIP

Have client flex the hip by bending the knee. Prop client's foot against your thigh. Interlace fingers and, using the thenar edge of the hand, hook into the quadriceps muscles. Apply a slow, deep slide from proximal attachment to distal.

Use the palms with a soft glide back to the proximal attachment and repeat three to five times.

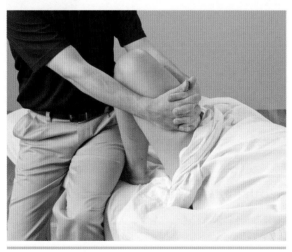

SEQUENCE 9-2 FIGURE 2

QUADRICEPS SEQUENCE

FRICTION

Apply friction to the ligaments of the knee. Apply friction around the patella, the medial and lateral collateral ligaments, and the patellar ligament and tendon at its attachment point at the tibial tuberosity.

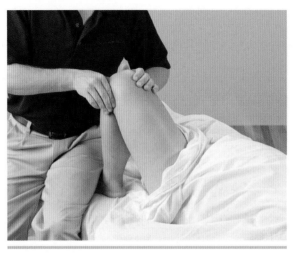

SEQUENCE 9-2 FIGURE 3

BALANCE THE THIGH

Apply deep slides and stretching to the hamstrings to balance the thigh.

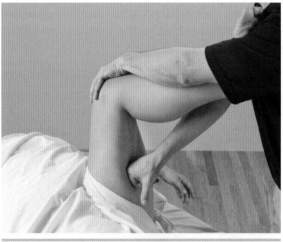

SEQUENCE 9-2 FIGURE 4

SEQUENCE 9-3

WARM UP TISSUES

Use pétrissage, deep slides, and stripping strokes to warm the tissues of the posterior hip.

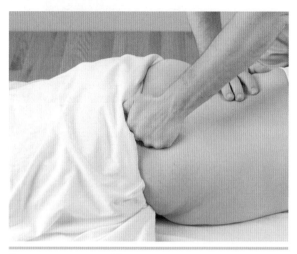

SEQUENCE 9-3 FIGURE 1

FRICTION

Apply multidirectional friction to all attachment points around the greater trochanter of the femur.

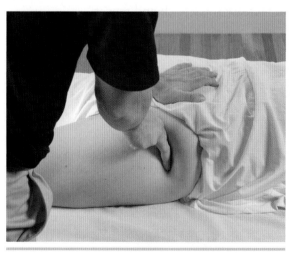

SEQUENCE 9-3 FIGURE 2

TRIGGER POINTS AND ROM

Apply compression to hypersensitive areas and flex the knee. Internally and externally rotate the hip.

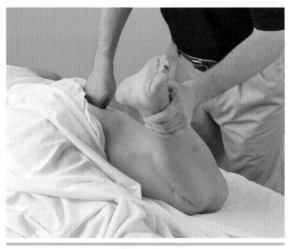

SEQUENCE 9-3 FIGURE 3

ACCESSING THE DEEP LATERAL ROTATORS

Abduct and flex the hip so the client's leg is off the table. Place the client's leg on your thigh. This position allows easier access to the deep lateral rotators.

Apply compression and have the client actively contract the muscle by pushing against your thigh. Hold the contraction and release. Slide the knee toward the head of the table to increase the stretch and repeat.

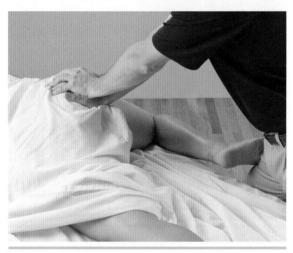

SEQUENCE 9-3 FIGURE 4

SEQUENCE 9-4

WARM UP TISSUES

Use pétrissage, deep slides, and broadening strokes to warm the tissues of the anterior thigh.

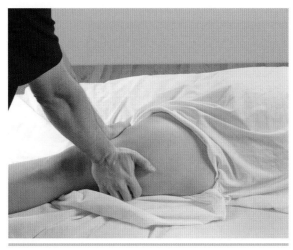

SEQUENCE 9-4 FIGURE 1

QUADRICEPS

Apply stripping strokes and friction to the vastus lateralis, vastus medialis, and rectus femoris. Address any trigger points in these muscles.

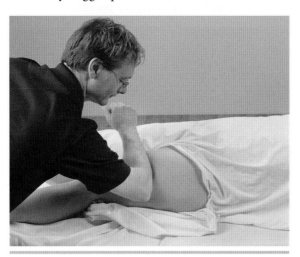

SEQUENCE 9-4 FIGURE 2

PATELLOFEMORAL SEQUENCE

FRICTION

Apply multidirectional friction to the quadriceps tendon above the knee. Apply cross-fiber friction to the patellar tendon superior to the tibial tuberosity.

Remove the bolster and straighten the leg. Carefully displace the patella laterally and apply multidirectional friction under the patella.

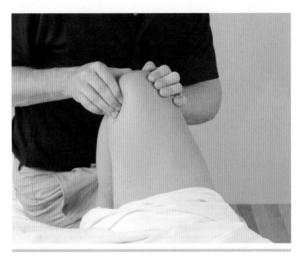

SEQUENCE 9-4 FIGURE 3

HAMSTRINGS

Use effleurage and pétrissage to warm the tissues of the hamstring. Apply stripping and broadening strokes and address any trigger points.

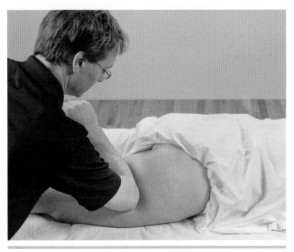

SEQUENCE 9-4 FIGURE 4

STRETCHING

Stretch the quadriceps by flexing the knee. The closer to the hip you can bring the foot, the better the stretch. If the client has the flexibility, you can extend the hip to place the stretch on the rectus femoris; however, our focus is on all quadriceps muscles.

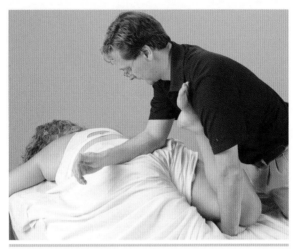

SEQUENCE 9-4 FIGURE 5

ILIOTIBIAL BAND DISORDERS SEQUENCE

SEQUENCE 9-5

WARM UP TISSUES

Use effleurage and pétrissage along the lateral thigh to warm the tissues.

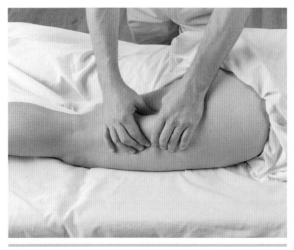

SEQUENCE 9-5 FIGURE 1

LENGTHENING

Apply deep slides moving from proximal to distal to encourage lengthening.
Move slowly with this technique, pausing at any area that is hypersensitive.
Apply myofascial techniques and stretching.

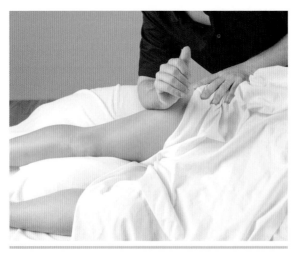

SEQUENCE 9-5 FIGURE 2

TENSOR FASCIA LATAE

Strip the TFL, moving from proximal to distal. Address any trigger points.

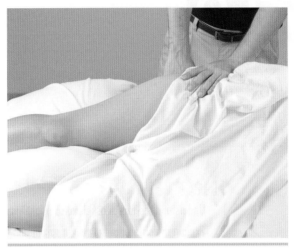

SEQUENCE 9-5 FIGURE 3

BALANCE THE THIGH

Apply effleurage, pétrissage, and stripping strokes to the adductor group.

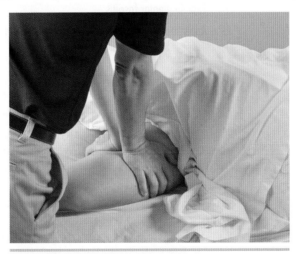

SEQUENCE 9-5 FIGURE 4

TFL, tensor fascia latae

CHAPTER 10

THE LEG

OUTLINE

KEY TERMS

acute compartment syndrome
body alignment
chronic compartment syndrome
compartment syndrome
compartments of the leg
edema
grades of sprains
grades of strains
gross movements
heel spur
locomotion
micromovements
microtears
muscle strain
periostitis
periosteum
plantar fascia
plantar fasciitis
sprains
shin splints
strain
tibial stress syndrome

OBJECTIVES

1   Understand the musculoskeletal components of the leg.
2   Explain the difference between a sprain and a strain.
3   Describe the grades of sprains and strains.
4   Explain shin splints and tibial stress syndromes.
5   Describe the compartments of the leg.
6   Understand the severity of compartment syndrome.
7   Explain plantar fasciitis.
8   Apply massage techniques for the leg and foot.

The leg and foot are constantly under pressure, literally. They are responsible for carrying our body weight and any additional loads over distances. The average person walks approximately 8,000 to 10,000 steps in a day. This is approximately 115,000 miles in a lifetime. Add sports and activities into the equation and one can see how the leg and foot are prone to several overuse and repetitive traumas.

The legs are used not only for **locomotion**, but also play a key role in balance and the minor adjustments necessary to maintain proper **body alignment** in a standing position and to maintain balance on uneven ground. Minor shifts in the alignment of the foot at the ankle create a chain of events that can lead to postural misalignments and compensation patterns that can lead to pain experienced in other areas.

ANATOMY OF THE LEG AND FOOT

The foot alone contains 26 bones, 33 joints, 107 ligaments, and 19 muscles (Figure 10-1). Add the tibia and fibula and the muscles of the leg, and you have a complex unit that allows for **gross movements** and **micromovements**. This chapter focuses on major musculature of the leg and its common injuries.

SPRAINED AND STRAINED ANKLES

It is important to understand the difference between sprain and strain injuries. The approach to care for these injuries varies and depends on the structure that is injured. A **strain** is an injury involving the musculotendinous unit.

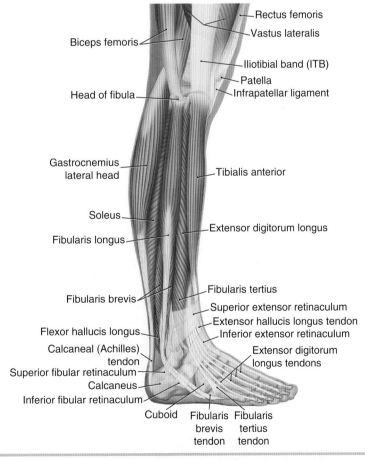

FIGURE 10-1 ■ Muscles of the leg and foot. (From Muscolino JE: *The muscle and bone palpation manual with trigger points, referral patterns, and stretching,* St Louis, 2009, Mosby.)

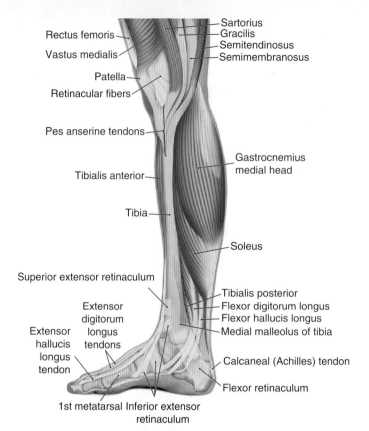

Sartorius
Rectus femoris
Gracilis
Semitendinosus
Vastus medialis
Semimembranosus
Patella
Retinacular fibers
Pes anserine tendons
Gastrocnemius medial head
Tibialis anterior
Tibia
Soleus
Superior extensor retinaculum
Tibialis posterior
Extensor digitorum longus
Flexor digitorum longus
Flexor hallucis longus
Extensor hallucis longus tendon
Extensor digitorum longus tendons
Medial malleolus of tibia
Calcaneal (Achilles) tendon
Flexor retinaculum
1st metatarsal   Inferior extensor retinaculum

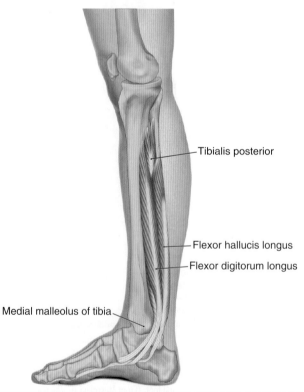

Tibialis posterior
Flexor hallucis longus
Flexor digitorum longus
Medial malleolus of tibia

FIGURE 10-1 ▦ cont'd.

These injuries are usually due to excessive contraction in the muscle or sudden elongation of the muscle. A strain happens in the muscle belly, the tendon, or at the musculotendinous junction. **Grades of strains** are categorized by the severity of the injury. Grade 1 strains are mild, and involve a minor stretch or tear. There is little loss in strength and mild discomfort. A grade 2 strain involves muscle fiber tears and a loss of strength. A more noticeable loss of strength and pain during activities is present. Grade 3 strains are the most severe. They involve a complete tear of the musculotendinous unit. This can occur at the bony attachment or in the muscle itself. The muscle bunches up and there is a noticeable change in the surface of the area. Those experiencing a grade 3 strain are unable to continue activities because of extreme pain and muscle weakness (Figure 10-2).

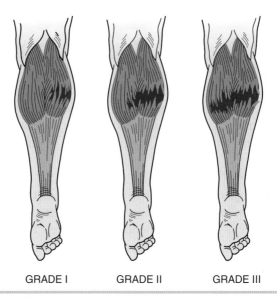

GRADE I   GRADE II   GRADE III

FIGURE 10-2 ■ **Muscle strain.** (From Salvo SG: *Massage therapy: principles and practice,* ed 2, Philadelphia, 2003, Saunders.)

Sprains occur when a ligament is overstretched or torn. These tears are most often caused by sudden twisting or shear force. Sprain and strain injuries present discomfort, swelling, heat, and some color changes depending on the severity. Ligament injuries also have an effect on the stability of the joint. **Grades of sprains** are categorized by the severity of the injury. In a grade 1 sprain the ligament is overstretched or has minor tearing. Although this may be slightly painful during activity, it does not affect activities of daily living and there is no loss in stability of the joint. A grade 2 sprain has ligamental tearing along with swelling and pain. There is often a snapping or popping sound at the moment of injury. This grade of injury shows some loss of stability and may appear to be hypermobile. In grade 3 sprains the ligament is completely ruptured. The joint is highly unstable and painful (Figure 10-3).

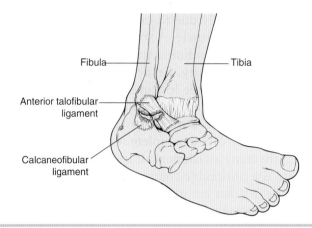

FIGURE 10-3 ■ Sprains. (From Frazier MS, Drzymkowski JW: *Essentials of human diseases and conditions,* ed 5, Philadelphia, 2013, Saunders.)

SHIN SPLINTS

Shin splints are a general term describing pain experienced on the anterior leg. When people complain of shin splints, they are usually referring to **tibial stress syndrome (TSS)**, **periostitis**, **acute compartment syndrome**, or **chronic compartment syndrome**. These pathologic conditions all have similar symptoms, which makes assessment challenging. Diagnosis should be confirmed by a medical doctor.

TIBIAL STRESS SYNDROME

TSS involves inflammation of the **periosteum** of the tibia. When people complain of shin splints or shin pain they may actually be complaining of TSS. Runners and gym-goers who spend most of their time on the treadmill are the leading groups who have complaints of this syndrome.

This condition is not due to muscular stress or trauma. TSS is actually a biomechanical disorder. The impact of running along with overpronation and poor support from the footwear creates pain on the anterior tibial surface (Figure 10-4). Most cases of TSS correct themselves with the addition of arch support and shoes that help prevent rotation of the tibia during activity (Sequence 10-1).

PERIOSTITIS

Periostitis is an inflammation of the periosteum or the fascia that surrounds the bone. The periosteum plays an important role, serving as an attachment for the muscles. The most common muscles involved with periostitis are the tibialis anterior, tibialis posterior, and the soleus. As these muscles begin to tighten and increase tension on the tibial periosteum, **microtears** may occur and the muscle may start to pull away from the bone. This ripping, repairing, and development of scar tissue is what gives the characteristic bumps and pitting of the tibial surface. Addressing the restrictions of the anterior and posterior tibialis muscles assists in the creation of healthy scar tissue and mobility of the tissues. The soleus muscle is another important muscle to understand when working with periostitis. Restrictions in the soleus can cause the interosseous membrane between the tibia and fibula to bind and restrict.

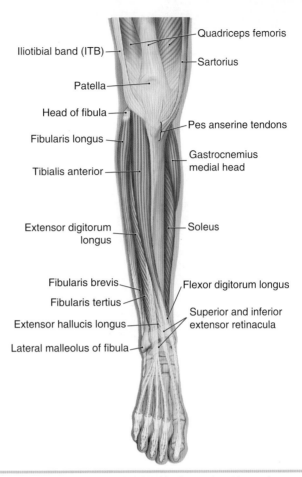

Iliotibial band (ITB)

Patella

Head of fibula

Fibularis longus

Tibialis anterior

Extensor digitorum
longus

Fibularis brevis

Fibularis tertius

Extensor hallucis longus

Lateral malleolus of fibula

Quadriceps femoris

Sartorius

Pes anserine tendons

Gastrocnemius
medial head

Soleus

Flexor digitorum longus

Superior and inferior
extensor retinacula

FIGURE 10-4 ■ Tibial stress syndrome. (From Muscolino JE: *The muscle and bone palpation manual with trigger points, referral patterns, and stretching,* St Louis, 2009, Mosby.)

COMPARTMENT SYNDROME

Compartment syndromes occur when the muscles of the leg engorge with blood and other fluids to the point at which circulation is impeded and the fluids cannot drain appropriately. The fascia in this area is thicker, with a higher tensile strength that does not allow it to expand easily. **Edema** and fluid retention increase the pressure in this area, which compresses the veins. This compression impedes the draining of the fluids, which in extreme cases can result in tissue death. Tissue death can take place in as little as 6-12 hours after injury. Compartment syndromes need to be assessed and treated by medical professionals as soon as possible.

There are four **compartments of the leg** which are susceptible to compartment syndromes: anterior, lateral, superficial posterior, and deep posterior (Figure 10-5). The anterior compartment is on the anterior and slightly lateral aspect of the leg between the tibia and fibula. This houses the tibialis anterior, extensor hallucis longus, extensor digitorum longus, and the peroneus (fibularis) tertius. The lateral compartment is found on the lateral aspect of the leg containing the peroneus (fibularis) longus and brevis. The superficial posterior compartment includes the gastrocnemius, soleus, and plantaris muscles. The deep posterior compartment is the hardest to access and is the compartment most

Text continued on p. 166

SHIN SPLINTS SEQUENCE

SEQUENCE 10-1

WARM UP TISSUES

Use myofascial release, pétrissage, and broadening strokes to warm up the tissues of the anterior leg.

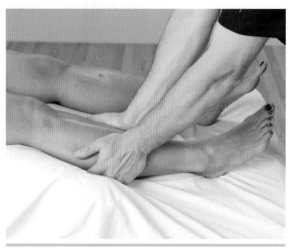

SEQUENCE 10-1 FIGURE 1

TIBIALIS ANTERIOR

Apply cross-fiber strokes moving from medial to lateral along the tibialis anterior. Address hypersensitive areas with trigger-point therapy and pin and stretch. Use deep longitudinal strokes and myofascial release along the medial border of the tibia.

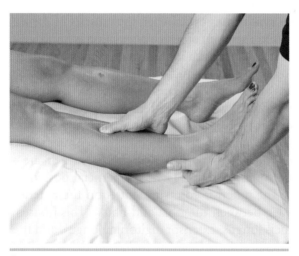

SEQUENCE 10-1 FIGURE 2

FRICTION TECHNIQUES
Apply multidirectional friction to the tendons of the dorsiflexors.

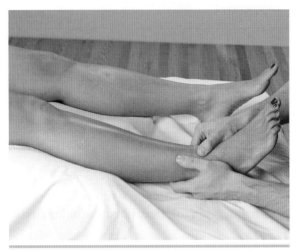

SEQUENCE 10-1 FIGURE 3

STRETCHING
Plantar-flex the foot to stretch the dorsiflexors of the foot.

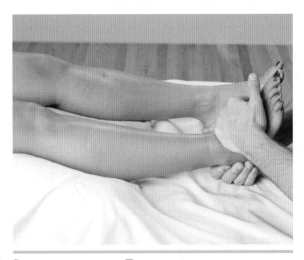

SEQUENCE 10-1 FIGURE 4

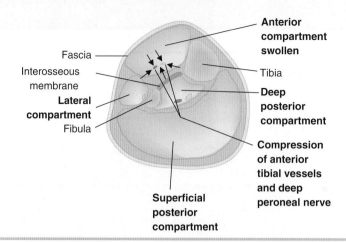

Anterior
compartment
swollen

Fascia

Interosseous
membrane

**Lateral
compartment**

Fibula

Tibia

**Deep
posterior
compartment**

**Compression
of anterior
tibial vessels
and deep
peroneal nerve**

**Superficial
posterior
compartment**

FIGURE 10-5 ■ Compartment syndrome. (From Black JM, Hawks JH, Keene AM: *Medical-surgical nursing: clinical management for positive outcomes,* ed 7, Philadelphia, 2005, Saunders.)

often involved in acute compartment syndrome cases. This compartment is around the flexor hallucis longus, flexor digitorum longus, and tibialis posterior.

Acute Compartment Syndrome

As a sudden-onset disorder, acute compartment syndrome is a serious disorder that often requires surgical intervention. Most cases of acute compartment syndrome are due to trauma to the leg from a fracture, break, or bleeding in the compartments of the leg. Because onset is sudden, massage is contraindicated. Acute compartment syndrome is a serious injury and can cause tissue death and possibly loss of the limb; immediate medical treatment is the only option.

Chronic Compartment Syndrome

Chronic compartment syndrome involves an increase in compartment pressure through muscle hypertrophy, increased fluids, and compromised drainage of the area. Unlike the acute version, chronic compartment syndrome is mostly caused by exercise and strenuous activity. Common complaints from people with chronic compartment syndrome include a feeling of tightness and swelling in the leg, numbness, limited movement in the foot, and pain. In most cases, symptoms disappear shortly after activity is stopped. This form of compartment syndrome is most commonly addressed with changes in the exercise program, footwear, or orthopedic inserts.

MASSAGE APPROACH TO THE LEG

When working with any of the shin splint–type injuries, it is important to remember that these are not muscular disorders. Shin splints, chronic compartment syndrome, and periostitis are connective-tissue disorders, and myofascial release techniques are the best approach.

Hypertonic muscles may be present while working on the leg. Using compressive techniques along with kneading and muscle squeezing are appropriate approaches for the musculature of the leg. A focus on strokes that encourage drainage and encourage blood flow help remove the edema and pooling of other fluids (Sequence 10-2).

SEQUENCE 10-2

SUPINE

Warm Up Tissues

Use myofascial release, pétrissage, and broadening strokes to warm up the tissues of the anterior leg.

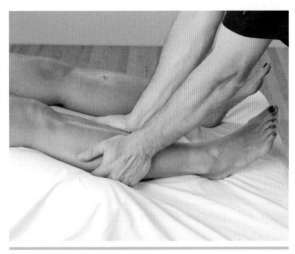

SEQUENCE 10-2 FIGURE 1

TIBIALIS ANTERIOR

Apply cross-fiber strokes moving from medial to lateral along the tibialis anterior. Address hypersensitive areas with trigger-point therapy and pin and stretch.

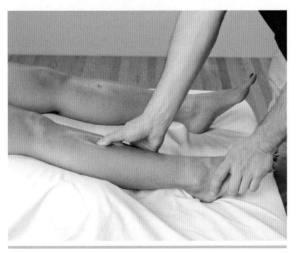

SEQUENCE 10-2 FIGURE 2

PERONEUS (FIBULARIS) MUSCLES

Apply cross-fiber strokes moving from medial to lateral along the peroneus muscles. Perform deep longitudinal strokes. Address hypersensitive areas with trigger point therapy and pin and stretch.

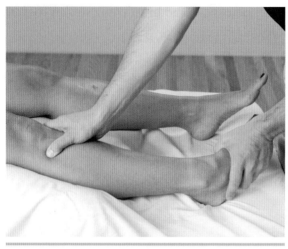

SEQUENCE 10-2 FIGURE 3

ANKLE MOBILIZATIONS

Move the ankle throughout its full range of motion. In its neutral position apply a slow consistent pull to traction the ankle.

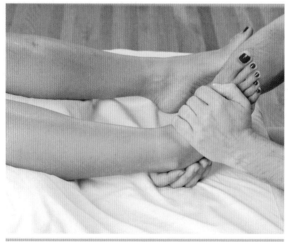

SEQUENCE 10-2 FIGURE 4

TRANSITION STROKES

Finish the anterior leg with effleurage strokes to encourage venous return.

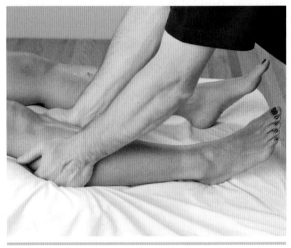

SEQUENCE 10-2 FIGURE 5

PRONE

Warm Up Tissues

Use myofascial release, pétrissage, and broadening strokes to warm up the tissues of the posterior leg.

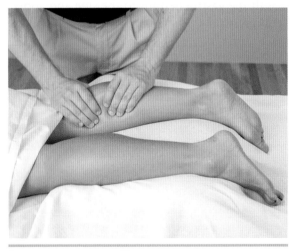

SEQUENCE 10-2 FIGURE 6

GASTROCNEMIUS

Apply deep longitudinal strokes and stripping strokes. Use compression strokes to address hypertonic areas. Add range of motion with the compression and longitudinal strokes to elongate the muscles.

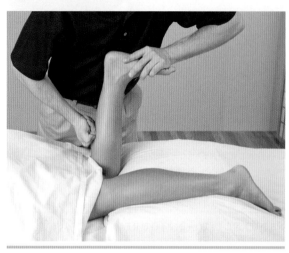

SEQUENCE 10-2 FIGURE 7

SOLEUS

The soleus muscle can be accessed on the medial and lateral sides of the leg under the gastrocnemius. Shift the gastrocnemius to the side and apply deep longitudinal strokes and digital compression.

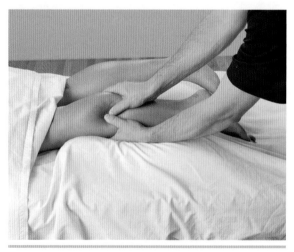

SEQUENCE 10-2 FIGURE 8

TENDONS AND LIGAMENTS OF THE ANKLE

Apply multidirectional friction to the ligaments of the ankle and the Achilles tendon.

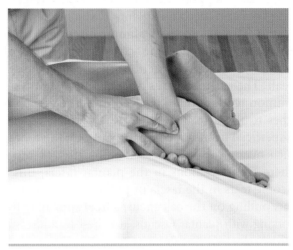

SEQUENCE 10-2 FIGURE 9

FINISHING

Finish the sequence with muscle-squeezing and effleurage to encourage venous return.

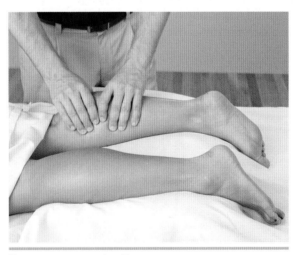

SEQUENCE 10-2 FIGURE 10

PLANTAR FASCIITIS

The **plantar fascia** is a thick band of connective tissue that covers the tarsals and metatarsals on the bottom of the foot. This band extends from the calcaneus to the heads of the five metatarsals. The plantar fascia acts like a rubber band to create tension, which maintains the arch of the foot while allowing some stretch during walking to help support the body and balance (Figure 10-6).

The plantar fascia can become inflamed, which often results in pain and difficulty in walking. This is known as **plantar fasciitis**. Risk factors such as high arches, flat feet, running, and extreme activity play a role in plantar fasciitis. One of the contributing factors is restrictions in the superficial posterior compartment of the calf. The gastrocnemius, soleus, and plantaris all merge together to form one common tendon, often referred to as the *Achilles tendon*. The Achilles tendon attaches to the calcaneus where the plantar fascia begins. The restrictions in the superficial posterior compartment pull the foot into a plantar-flexed position, which may result in increased elongation of the plantar fascia when walking. If there are restrictions in the plantar fascia, this increased pull may cause microscopic tears in the fascia or pull the fascia away from the calcaneus. Because of this pulling on the calcaneus, a **heel spur** may form.

When working with plantar fasciitis, it is best to address all areas that lead to the pain and discomfort. Although many may recommend the application of ice to control the swelling, cold causes the fascia to thicken and become less pliable. Warm foot baths and heat along with the use of foot rollers help soften the fascia. Massage therapy can aid in the stretching and elongation potential of the calf muscles and the plantar fascia. Working the trigger points and hypertonicity of the soleus and the gastrocnemius are equally important. Active and resistive range of motion along with deep slides has also shown benefits. Stripping with the knuckles of the plantar fascia can be painful, especially if the client is hypersensitive at the time of the session; however, a deeper connective tissue approach is effective (Sequence 10-3).

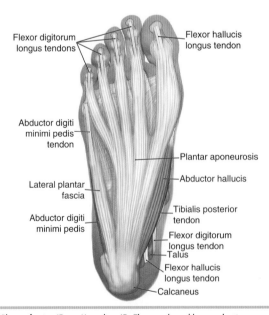

FIGURE 10-6 ■ Plantar fascia. (From Muscolino JE: *The muscle and bone palpation manual with trigger points, referral patterns, and stretching,* St Louis, 2009, Mosby.)

SEQUENCE 10-3

WARM UP TISSUES

Use myofascial release, pétrissage, and broadening strokes to warm up the tissues of the posterior leg.

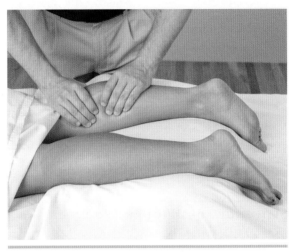

SEQUENCE 10-3 FIGURE 1

GASTROCNEMIUS

Apply deep longitudinal slides to the gastrocnemius and the Achilles tendon. Address the trigger points found in the gastrocnemius, soleus, and plantaris muscles.

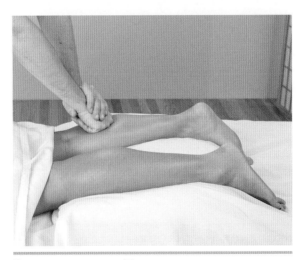

SEQUENCE 10-3 FIGURE 2

PLANTAR FASCIITIS SEQUENCE

FRICTION

Apply cross-fiber friction to the Achilles tendon at its attachment on the calcaneus.

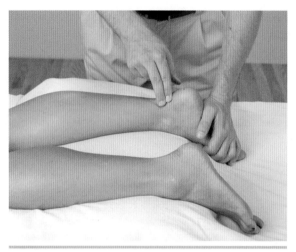

SEQUENCE 10-3 FIGURE 3

PLANTAR FASCIA

Use effleurage and digital stripping strokes to warm the plantar fascia. Apply deep longitudinal strokes from the calcaneus to the distal metatarsals. Use your other hand to support the foot. Broaden the plantar surface by starting at the midline and stroking to the sides.

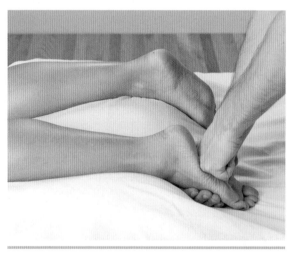

SEQUENCE 10-3 FIGURE 4

STRETCHING

End the sequence with stretching to the gastrocnemius and plantar surface of the foot.

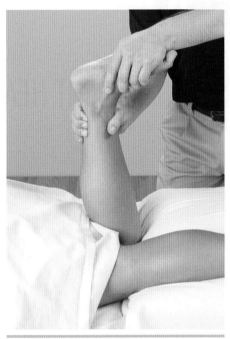

SEQUENCE 10–4 FIGURE 5

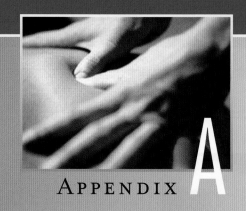

APPENDIX A

FIRST-TIME CLIENT HEALTH HISTORY

Client Information

Name _____ Phone (___)_____ DOB _____

Address _____ City _____ State _____ Zip _____

Email _____

Referred By _____ Phone (___) _____

In Case Of Emergency _____ Phone (___) _____

General & Medical Information

Occupation _____ Male ___ Female ___ Physician _____

Health Insurance Carrier _____

Please take a moment to carefully read the following information and sign where indicated. If you have a specific medical condition or specific symptoms, massage/bodywork may be contraindicated. A referral from your primary care provider may be required prior to service being provided.

Yes No   Have you ever experienced a professional massage or bodywork session? How recently?_____

If you answer "yes" to any of the following questions, please explain as clearly as possible.

Yes No   Do you frequently suffer from stress?
Yes No   Do you have diabetes?
Yes No   Do you experience frequent headaches?
Yes No   Are you pregnant?
Yes No   Do you suffer from arthritis?
Yes No   Are you wearing contact lenses?
Yes No   Are you wearing dentures?
Yes No   Do you have high blood pressure?
Yes No   If "yes" to previous question, are you taking medication for this?
Yes No   Do you suffer from epilepsy or seizures?
Yes No   Do you suffer from joint swelling?
Yes No   Do you have varicose veins?
Yes No   Do you have any contagious diseases?
Yes No   Do you have osteoporosis?
Yes No   Do you have any allergies?
Yes No   Do you bruise easily?

Yes No   Have you had any broken bones in the past two years?
Yes No   Have you been in an accident or suffered any injuries in the past two years?
Yes No   Do you have tension or soreness in a specific area? Please specify _____
_____

Yes No   Do you have cardiac or circulatory problems?
Yes No   Do you suffer from back pain?
Yes No   Do you have numbness or stabbing pains anywhere?
Yes No   Are you very sensitive to touch or pressure in any area?
Yes No   Have you ever had surgery? Explain below.
Yes No   Do you have any other medical condition, or are you taking any medications I should know about?

Comments _____
_____

I understand that the massage/bodywork I receive is provided for the basic purpose of relaxation and relief of muscular tension. If I experience any pain or discomfort during this session, I will immediately inform the practitioner so that the pressure and/or strokes may be adjusted to my level of comfort. I further understand that massage or bodywork should not be construed as a substitute for medical examination, diagnosis, or treatment and that I should see a physician, chiropractor, or other qualified medical specialist for any mental or physical ailment of which I am aware. I understand that massage/bodywork practitioners are not qualified to perform spinal or skeletal adjustments, diagnose, prescribe, or treat any physical or mental illness, and that nothing said in the course of the session given should be construed as such. Because massage/bodywork should not be performed under certain medical conditions, I affirm that I have stated all my known medical conditions and answered all questions honestly. I agree to keep the practitioner updated as to any changes in my medical profile and understand that there shall be no liability on the practitioner's part should I fail to do so. I also understand that any illicit or sexually suggestive remarks or advances made by me will result in immediate termination of the session, and I will be liable for payment of the scheduled appointment.

Client Signature _____ Date _____

Practitioner Signature _____ Date _____

Consent to Treatment of Minor: By my signature below, I hereby authorize (Company Name) to administer massage, bodywork, or somatic therapy techniques to my child or dependent as they deem necessary.

Signature of Parent or Guardian _____ Date _____

A-1 ▦ First-time client health history. (Courtesy Associated Bodywork & Massage Professionals.)

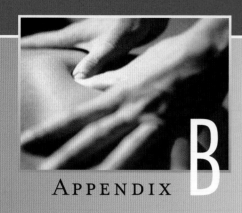

CLIENT INTAKE INFORMATION FORM

CLIENT INTAKE INFORMATION FORM

Name: _____ Date: _____

Address: _____ City: _____ State: _____ Zip: _____

Phone: (day) _____ (eve) _____ Date of Birth: _____

Occupation: _____ Employer: _____

Referred by: _____ Physician: _____

Previous experience with massage:

_____

Primary reason for appointment/areas of pain or tension:

_____

Emergency contact (name and number): _____

**Please mark (X) for all conditions that apply now. Put a (P) for past conditions,
an (F) for family history of illness.**

Pain Scale: minor-1   2   3   4   5   6   7   8   9   severe-10

___ headaches, migraines	___ chronic pain	___ fatigue
___ vision problems, contact lenses	___ muscle or joint pain	___ tension, stress
___ hearing problems, deafness	___ muscle, bone injuries	___ depression
___ injuries to face or head	___ numbness or tingling	___ sleep difficulties
___ sinus problems	___ sprains, strains	___ allergies, sensitivities
___ dental bridges, braces	___ arthritis, tendonitis	___ rashes, athletes foot
___ jaw pain, TMJ problems	___ cancer, tumors	___ infectious diseases
___ asthma or lung conditions	___ spinal column disorders	___ blood clots
___ constipation, diarrhea	___ diabetes	___ varicose veins
___ hernia	___ pregnancy	___ high/low blood pressure
___ birth control, IUD	___ heart, circulatory problems	
___ abdominal or digestive problems	___ other medical conditions not listed	

Explain any areas noted above:

_____

_____

Current medications, including aspirin, ibuprofen, herbs, supplements, etc.:

_____

_____

Surgeries: _____

Accidents: _____

Please list all forms and frequency of stress reduction activities, hobbies, exercise, or
sports participation: _____

_____

B-1 ■ Sample history form. This information is provided by the client. The key to completing the form is to ask questions. (From Fritz S: *Mosby's fundamentals of therapeutic massage,* ed 4, St Louis, 2009, Mosby.)

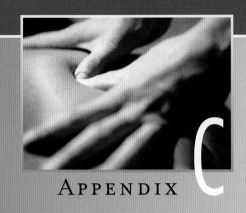

APPENDIX C

CLIENT INTAKE FORM

Client Intake Form

Name: _____

Address: _____

Telephone: (__)_____ Telephone: (__)_____

Email: _____

Date of birth: _____ Occupation: _____

Emergency contact: _____ Telephone: (__)_____

Previous massage experience: _____

Are you under medical supervision? _____

Regular physician: _____ Telephone: (__)_____

Referred by: _____

Check all that apply:

□ Allergies	□ Heart condition	□ Previous MVA/trauma
□ Arthritis	□ Infection	□ Ruptured/bulging disk
□ Blood clots	□ Infl ammation	□ Seizure disorders
□ Bruise easily	□ Kidney disorder	□ Stroke
□ Cancer	□ Medications affecting blood clotting	□ Recent surgery
□ Diabetes	□ Pregnancy	□ Varicose veins/thrombophlebitus

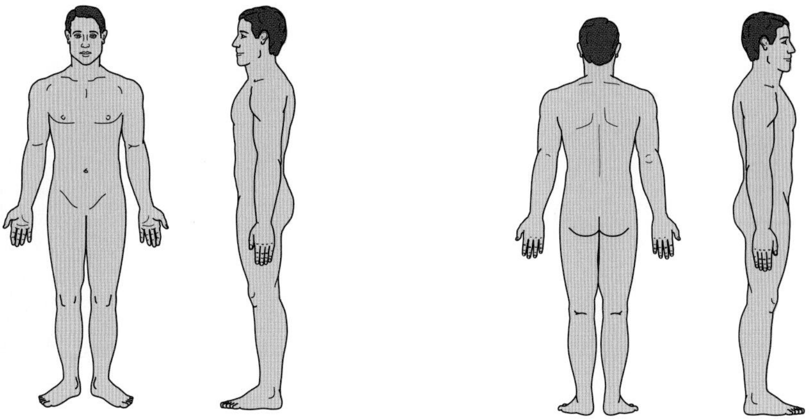

Identify your painful areas on these drawings using an X

Please briefly explain all checked items: _____

_____

_____

Signature: _____ Date: _____

C-1 ■ Client intake form. (From Salvo S: *Massage therapy: principles and practice,* ed 4, St Louis, 2012, Mosby.)

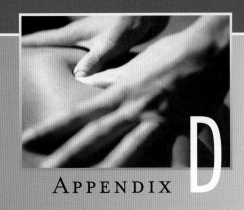

APPENDIX D

HEALTH HISTORY UPDATE

Health History Update

Client: _____ Date: _____

   1. Have there been any changes in your health since your last visit?

      _____

      _____

   2. Have you recently required other health services?_____

      If yes, nature of care _____

   3. Physician's name: _____

   4. Have you been hospitalized since your last visit? _____

      If yes, nature of problem _____

   5. Any new illnesses? _____

      _____

   6. Are you taking any medication(s) now? _____

  To treat: _____

  Name and dosage: _____

   7. Do you have any new allergies or reactions to any medications or drugs?

      _____

   8. Women only: Are you pregnant? _____ If yes, due date: _____

   9. Any other new diseases, conditions, or problems you think we should know about?

      _____

      _____

Client signature: _____

Massage therapist signature: _____

D-1 ■ Health history update.

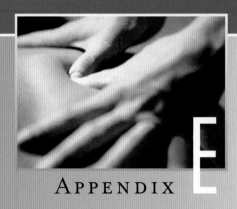

APPENDIX E

PERSONAL INFORMATION UPDATE

Personal Information Update

Name: _____ Date: _____

1. Has your name changed since your last visit here?   ☐ Yes   ☐ No

   If yes, what was the old name? _____

   What name do you use for insurance if different than above? _____

   _____

2. If you have a new or different address since your initial visit here, please indicate below:

   _____

   _____

   _____

   Please indicate if any apartment # or P.O. Box # _____

3. Has your marital status changed?   ☐ Yes   ☐ No

4. Has your telephone number changed?   ☐ Yes   ☐ No

   Please indicate your correct telephone number _____

5. Has your employment changed?   ☐ Yes   ☐ No

   Please indicate your new employer name and address:

   _____

   _____

   _____

New employer telephone # _____

6. Have you changed insurance companies?   ☐ Yes   ☐ No

   If yes, please indicate your new insurance carrier and address

   Primary _____   Secondary _____

   _____   _____

   _____   _____

   Group #_____   Group #_____

   Subscriber # _____   Subscriber # _____

7. Who is responsible for this bill? _____

8. Signature _____

Thank you for your assistance

E-1 ▦ Personal information update.

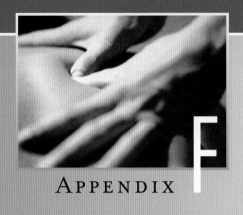

APPENDIX F

ASSESSMENT SHEET

MASSAGE ASSESSMENT/PHYSICAL OBSERVATION/PALPATION AND GAIT PRE ⟋ POST ⟋

Client Name: _____ Date: _____

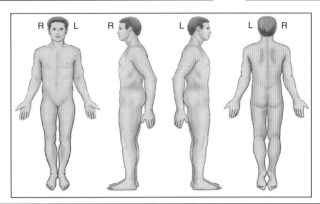

OBSERVATION & PALPATION		
ALIGNMENT	**RIBS**	**SCAPULA**
Chin in line with nose, sternal notch, navel	Even	Even
Other:	Springy	Move freely
HEAD	Other:	Other:
Tilted (L)	**ABDOMEN**	**CLAVICLES**
Tilted (R)	Firm and pliable	Level
Rotated (L)	Hard areas	Other:
Rotated (R)	Other:	**ARMS**
EYES	**WAIST**	Hang evenly (internal) (external)
Level	Level	(L) rotated ☐ medial ☐ lateral
Equally set in socket	Other:	(R) rotated ☐ medial ☐ lateral
Other:	**SPINE CURVES**	**ELBOWS**
EARS	Normal	Even ☐
Level	Other:	Other:
Other:	**GLUTEAL MUSCLE MASS**	**WRISTS**
SHOULDERS	Even	Even
Level	Other:	Other:
(R) high / (L) low	**ILIAC CREST**	**FINGERTIPS**
(L) high / (R) low	Level	Even
(L) rounded forward	Other:	Other:
(R) rounded forward	**KNEES**	**PATELLA**
Muscle development even	Even/symmetrical	(L) ☐ movable ☐ rigid
Other:	Other:	(R) ☐ movable ☐ rigid

F-1 ▦ A sample physical assessment form. This information is obtained by observing (looking and feeling) and measuring. The key to completing the form is to identify what is the same on the two sides of the body and what is different. (From Fritz S: *Mosby's fundamentals of therapeutic massage,* ed 4, St Louis, 2009, Mosby.)

ANKLES		TRUNK		LEGS	
Even		Remains vertical		Swing freely at hip	
Other:		Other:		Other:	
FEET		**SHOULDERS**		**KNEES**	
Mobile		Remain level		Flex and extend freely through stance and swing phase	
Other:		Rotate during walking		Other:	
ARCHES		Other:		**FEET**	
Even		**ARMS**		Heel strikes first at start of stance	
Other:		Motion is opposite leg swing		Plantar flexed at push-off	
TOES		Motion is even (L) and (R)		Foot clears floor during swing phase	
Straight		Other:		Other:	
Other:		(L) swings freely		**STEP**	
SKIN		(R) swings freely		Length is even	
Moves freely and resilient		Other:		Timing is even	
Pulls/restricted		**HIPS**		Other:	
Puffy/baggy		Remain level		**OVERALL**	
Other:		Other:		Rhythmic	
HEAD		Rotate during walking		Other:	
Remains steady/eyes forward		Other:			
Other:					

F-1 ▦ cont'd.

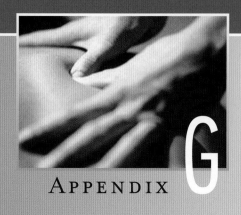

APPENDIX G

TREATMENT PLAN

TREATMENT PLAN

Client Name: _____

Choose One: ☐ Original plan   ☐ Reassessment date _____

Short-term client goals:
Quantitative: _____
Qualitative: _____

Long-term client goals:
_____
_____

Therapist objectives:
_____
_____

1) Frequency, 2) length, and 3) duration of visits:
1) _____   2) _____   3) _____

Progress measurements to be used: (Ex.— pain scale, range of motion, increased ability to perform function)
_____
_____

Dates of reassessment:
_____

Categories of massage methods to be used: (Ex.— general constitutional, stress reduction, circulatory, lymphatic, neuromuscular, connective tissue, neurochemical, etc.)
_____
_____

Additional notes:
_____
_____
_____

Client Signature: _____   Date: _____

Therapist Signature: _____   Date: _____

G-1 ▦ A sample form for a care/treatment plan. (From Fritz S: *Mosby's fundamentals of therapeutic massage,* ed 4, St Louis, 2009, Mosby.)

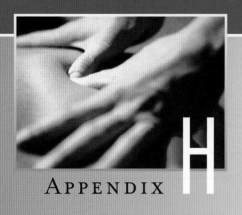

APPENDIX H

INITIAL ASSESSMENT

Initial Assessment

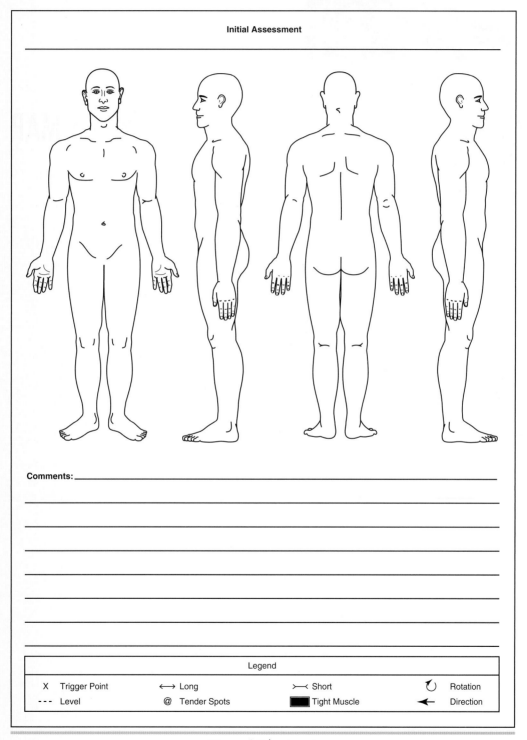

Comments: _____

_____
_____
_____
_____
_____
_____
_____
_____

Legend			
X Trigger Point	⟷ Long	⟩——⟨ Short	↻ Rotation
- - - Level	@ Tender Spots	▨ Tight Muscle	← Direction

H-1 ▥ Initial assessment.

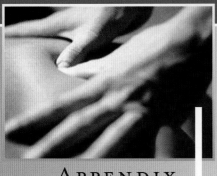

APPENDIX

BODY MAP

Body Map

Client: _____   Date: _____

Observations/Recommendations: _____

_____

Range of Motion: _____%   Pain Threshold: ❏ High   ❏ Low

Client Preferences: _____

Contraindications: _____

Indications: _____

Arm
❏ Biceps/Tricep Supinator
❏ Brachialis
❏ Coracobrachialis
❏ Deltoids: Ant/Lat/Post
❏ Pronator Teres

Hip/Leg
❏ Add Long/Brev Mag
❏ Biceps Femoris
❏ Gemellus Sup/Inf
❏ Gluteus Max/Med/Min
❏ Obturator Int/Ext
❏ Pectineus
❏ Piriformis
❏ Psoas Major/Illacus
❏ Quadratus Femoris
❏ Rectus Femoris
❏ Sacrospinalis
❏ Sartorius/Gracilis
❏ Semi-Tend/Membranosus
❏ Tensor Fasiae Latae
❏ Trochanteric
❏ Vastus Int/Med/Lat

Neck
❏ Scalenes Anter/Med/Post
❏ Splenus Capitus
❏ Splenus Cervicus
❏ Sternocleidomastoid
❏ Supra Infra Hyoids

Chest
❏ Diaphragm
❏ Ext/Int Oblique
❏ Intercostals
❏ Pectoralis Major/Minor
❏ Rectus Abdominis
❏ Ribs
❏ Serratus Anterior
❏ Subclavius
❏ Transverse Abdominis

Foot
❏ Abd/Add Hallucis Brev
❏ Abductor Digiti Brevis
❏ Dors/Plan Interossei
❏ Flexor Digiti Minimi Brevis
❏ Flexor Digitorum Brevis
❏ Flexor Hallucis Brevis
❏ Lumbricals
❏ Quadratus Plantae
❏ Retrocalcaneal

Lower Leg
❏ Flex/Ext Digitorum Long/BR
❏ Flex/Ext Hallucis Long
❏ Gastrocnemius
❏ Peroneus Tert/Brev/Lon
❏ Plantaris/Popliteus
❏ Soleus
❏ Tibialis Post/Ant

Back
❏ Erector Spinae
❏ Iliocostalis
❏ Infraspinatus
❏ Interspinalis
❏ Intertransversarii
❏ Latissimus Dorsi
❏ Levator Scapula
❏ Longissimum
❏ Multifidus Rotatores
❏ Quadratus Lumborum
❏ Rhomboids: Major/Minor
❏ Serratus Post/Sup/Inf
❏ Spinalis/Semispinalis
❏ Subscapularis
❏ Supraspinatus
❏ Teres Major/Minor
❏ Trapezius

Head
❏ Auricularis Post/Sup
❏ Buccinator
❏ Masseter
❏ Orbicularis Oris/Occuli
❏ Pterygoid Med/Lat
❏ Transverse Nuchae
❏ Temporalis

I-I ▦ Body map. (Courtesy Associated Bodywork & Massage Professionals.)

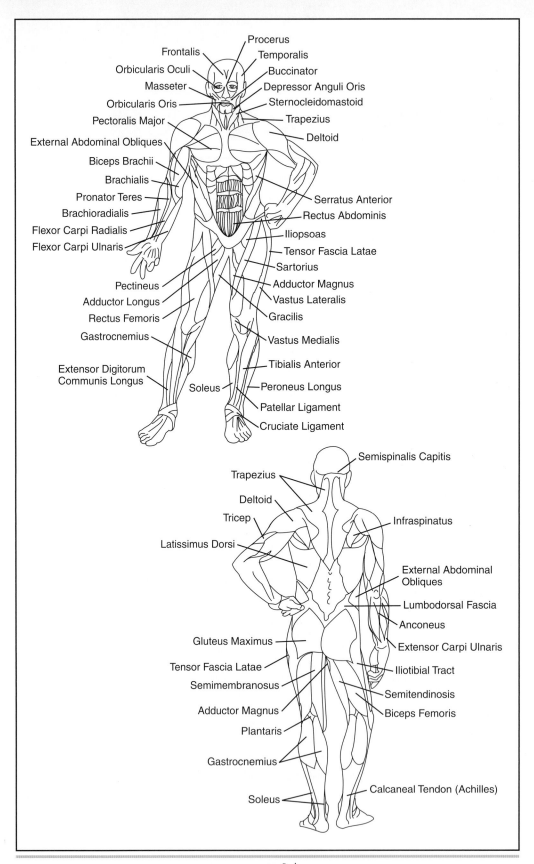

Procerus
Frontalis
Temporalis
Orbicularis Oculi
Buccinator
Masseter
Depressor Anguli Oris
Orbicularis Oris
Sternocleidomastoid
Pectoralis Major
Trapezius
External Abdominal Obliques
Deltoid
Biceps Brachii
Brachialis
Pronator Teres
Serratus Anterior
Brachioradialis
Rectus Abdominis
Flexor Carpi Radialis
Iliopsoas
Flexor Carpi Ulnaris
Tensor Fascia Latae
Sartorius
Pectineus
Adductor Magnus
Adductor Longus
Vastus Lateralis
Rectus Femoris
Gracilis
Gastrocnemius
Vastus Medialis
Tibialis Anterior
Extensor Digitorum
Communis Longus
Soleus
Peroneus Longus
Patellar Ligament
Cruciate Ligament

Semispinalis Capitis
Trapezius
Deltoid
Tricep
Infraspinatus
Latissimus Dorsi
External Abdominal
Obliques
Lumbodorsal Fascia
Anconeus
Gluteus Maximus
Extensor Carpi Ulnaris
Tensor Fascia Latae
Iliotibial Tract
Semimembranosus
Semitendinosis
Adductor Magnus
Biceps Femoris
Plantaris
Gastrocnemius
Calcaneal Tendon (Achilles)
Soleus

I-I ■ cont'd Body map.

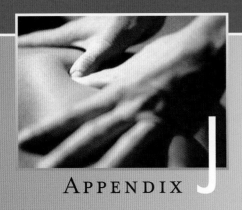

APPENDIX J

HIPAA FORM

NOTICE OF PRIVACY PRACTICES FOR PROTECTED HEALTH INFORMATION

Law requires the privacy of your health information be maintained and that you are provided this notice of the legal duties and privacy practices with respect to your health information. Other than the uses and disclosures we described below, your health information will not be sold or provided to any outside marketing organization. We must abide by the terms of this notice and we reserve the right to change the terms of this privacy notice. If a change is made, it will apply for all of your health information in our files, and you will be notified in writing.

HOW INFORMATION ABOUT YOU MAY BE USED AND DISCLOSED AND HOW YOU CAN GET ACCESS TO THIS INFORMATION.

USES AND DISCLOSURES

Here are examples of use and disclosure of your health care information:

1. We may have to disclose your health information to another health care provider, or a hospital, etc., if it is necessary to refer you to them for the diagnosis, assessment, or treatment of your health condition.
2. We may have to disclose your session records and your billing records to another party (i.e., your insurance company), if they are potentially responsible for the payment of your services.
3. We may need to use any information in your file for quality control purposes or any other administrative purposes to run this practice.
4. We may need to use your name, address, phone number, and your records to contact you to provide appointment reminder calls, recall postcards, Welcome and Thank You cards, information about alternative therapies, or other related information that may be of interest to you. If you are not at home to receive an appointment reminder, a message will be left on your answering machine.

YOUR RIGHT TO LIMIT USES OR DISCLOSURES

You have the right to request that we do not disclose your information to specific individuals, companies, or organizations. Any restrictions should be requested in writing. We are not required to honor these requests. If we agree with your restrictions, the restriction is binding on us.

PERMITTED USES AND DISCLOSURES WITHOUT YOUR CONSENT OR AUTHORIZATION

Under federal law, we are also permitted or required to use or disclose your information without your consent or authorization in the following circumstances:

1. We are providing services to you based on the orders (referral) of a health care provider.
2. We provide services to you in an emergency and are unable to obtain your consent after attempting to do so.
3. If there are substantial barriers to communicating with you, but in our professional judgment we believe that you intend for us to provide care.

REVOKING YOUR AUTHORIZATION

You may revoke your authorization to us at any time in writing. There are two circumstances under which we will not be able to honor your revocation request:

1. If your information has been released prior to your request to revoke your authorization.
2. If you were required to give your authorization as a condition of obtaining insurance, the insurance company may have a right to your information if they decide to contest any of your claims.

CONFIDENTIAL COMMUNICATION

We will attempt to accommodate any reasonable written request regarding your contact information that has been provided by you.

J-1 ▦ Health Insurance Portability and Accountability Act form.

AMENDING YOUR HEALTH INFORMATION

You have the right to request that we amend your health information for seven years from the date that the record was created or as long as the information remains in our files. We require a written request to amend your records that includes a valid reason to support the change. We have the right to refuse your request.

INSPECTING/COPYING YOUR HEALTH INFORMATION

You have the right to inspect your files while in our office and/or have a copy made for you. The information is available up to seven years from the date that the record was created.

Your request to inspect or obtain a copy of the file must be in writing. There will be a charge of $.20 per page copied.

ACCOUNTING OF DISCLOSURES OF YOUR RECORDS

You have the right to request an accounting of any disclosures (not listed below) made of your information for six years prior to the date of your request. The request must be in writing. The accounting will exclude the following disclosures:

Required for your session, to obtain payment for services, to run our practice, and/or made to you. Necessary to maintain a directory of the individuals in our facility or to individuals involved in your care. For national security, intelligence purposes, or law enforcement officers.

That were made prior to the effective date of the HIPAA privacy law (April 14, 2003).

We will provide the first accounting within a 12-month period without any charge, but any additional requests will be charged a fee. When you make your request we will tell you the amount of the fee and you will have the opportunity to withdraw or modify your request

RE-DISCLOSURE

We cannot control the actions of others to whom we have released your information for further treatment. Information that we use or disclose may be subject to re-disclosure by these individuals/facilities and may no longer be protected by the federal privacy rules.

COMPLAINTS

You may complain to us or to the Secretary for Health and Human Services if you feel that we have violated your privacy rights. We respect your right to file a complaint and will not take any action against you if you file a complaint. Written comments should be addressed to our office address or Secretary for Health and Human Services, 200 Independence Ave. SW, Room 509F, HHH Bldg. Washington, DC 20201.

This notice effective as of April 14, 2003. This notice will expire six years after the date upon which the record was created. By signing below, I acknowledge that I was given the opportunity to read and ask questions.

I, _____, give my permission for you to leave any information for me and use your name/clinic name at the following:

Home phone _____   Work phone _____

Cell phone _____   Fax _____

Client Name (Printed) _____   Date _____

Client Signature _____   Authorized Staff Person_____

Personal Representative (Printed) _____

Personal Representative Signature_____

Description of personal representative's authority to act for the client. _____

_____

J-1 ▪ cont'd. HIPAA form.

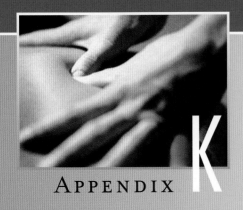

APPENDIX K

SOAP NOTES

SESSION NOTES
SOAP CHARTING FORM

Client Name: _____ Date: _____

Practitioner Name: _____

S ubjective **CLIENT STATUS**

- **Information from client, referral source, or reference books:**

1) Current conditions/changes from last session: _____

_____

_____

_____

O bjective **CONTENT OF SESSION**

- **Generate goal (possibilities) from analysis of information in <u>client status</u>.**

1) Information from <u>assessment</u> (physical, gait, palpation, muscle testing):

_____

_____

2) Goals worked on this session. (Base information on client status this session and goals previously established
   in Treatment Plan):

_____

_____

A nalysis **RESULTS**

- **Analyze results of session in relationship to what was done and how this relates to the session goals. (This is
  based on <u>cause</u> and <u>effect</u> of methods used and the effects on the persons involved).**

1) What was <u>done</u> this session:

_____

_____

2) What worked/what didn't: (Based on measurable and objective Post Assessment)

_____

_____

_____

P lan **PLAN:** Plans for next session, what client will work on, what next massage will reassess and continue to assess: _____

_____

_____

CLIENT COMMENTS:

_____

Time In: _____ Time Out: _____

Therapist signature: _____

K-1 ■ A SOAP charting form modified for student learning. The key to completing the form is to answer the questions based on what happened during the massage. (From Fritz S: *Mosby's Fundamentals of Therapeutic Massage,* ed 4, St Louis, 2009, Mosby.)

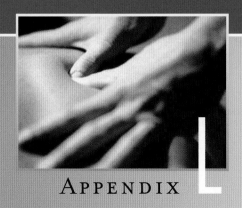

APPENDIX L

SOAP NOTES (short)

Client Name _____

Session Number ___ and ___ Total Hours

_____

S

O

A

P

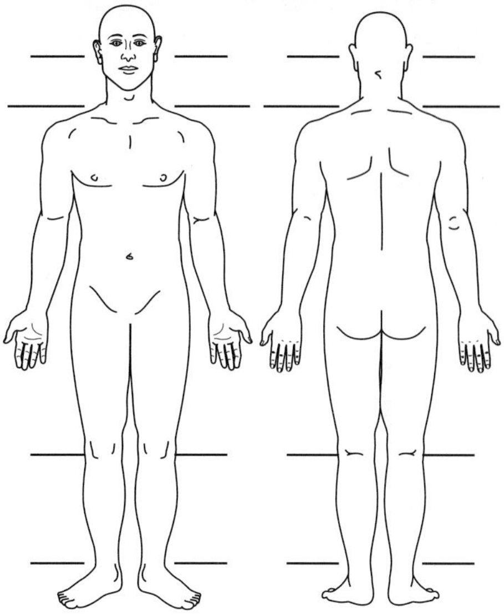

Provider Signature _____ Date _____

S

O

A

P

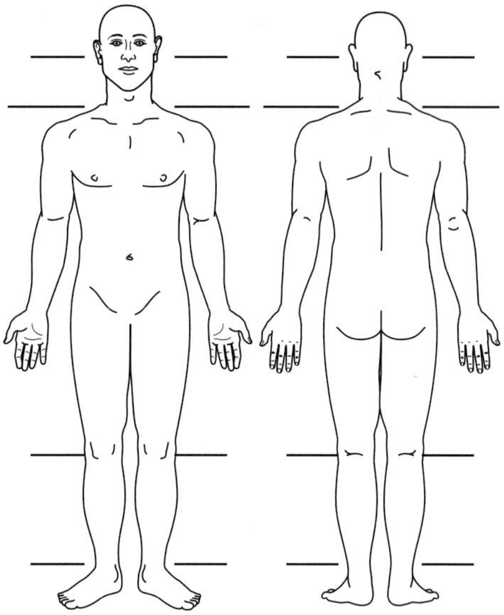

Provider Signature _____ Date _____

Legend: ℮ TP   ● TeP   ○ Ⓟ   ✳ Infl   ≡ HT   ≈ SP

         × Adh   ≷ Numb   ↻ rot   ╱ elev   ⊶ Short   ↔ Long

L-I ▦ SOAP notes (short).

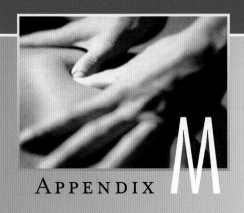

APPENDIX M

SOAP NOTES (detailed)

Client Name: _____ Date: _____

Subjective:

    Location:

    Onset:

    Characteristics:

    Quality:

    Severity:

    Additional symptoms:

    Treatments (past):

Objective:

    Postural assessment:

    Gait assessment:

    Functional assessment:

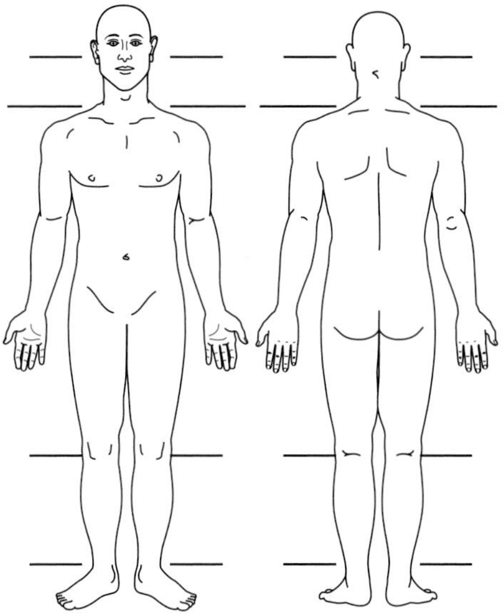

Assessments:

    Duration:

    Modalities used:

    Changes:

Plan:

    Homework:

    Short term:

    Long term:

M–I ▦ SOAP notes (detailed).

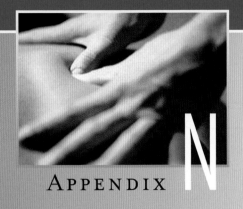

APPENDIX N

CARE NOTES

Client Name: _____ Date: _____

Duration of Session: _____

Condition:

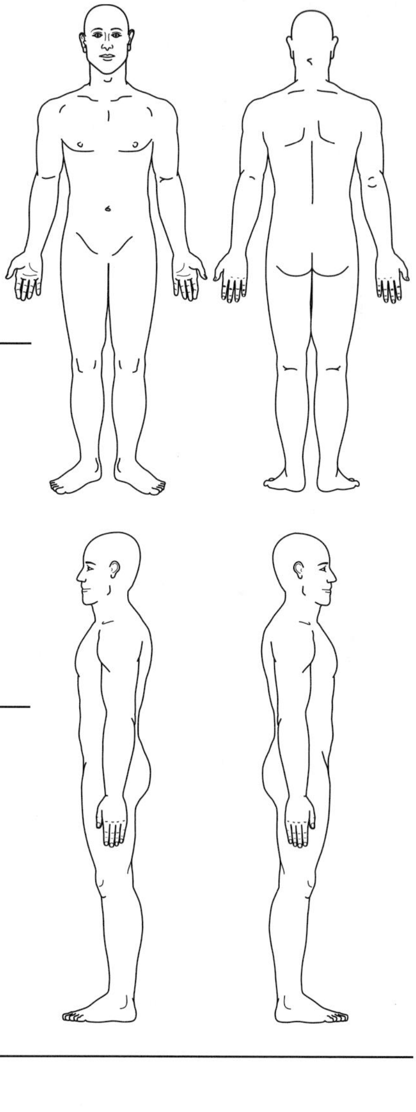

Action:

Response:

Evaluation:

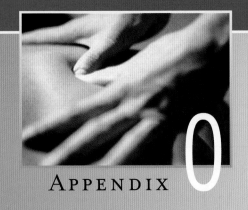

APPENDIX 0

APIE NOTES

```
                                              APIE Notes

   Client Name: _____  Date: _____

   A:




   P:




   I:




   E:




   Therapist's signature: _____


   Legend: A=Assessment   P=Plan of care   I=Implementation   E=Evaluation
```

O-1 ▦ APIE notes. (Modified from Salvo S: *Massage therapy: principles and practice,* ed 3, St Louis, 2008, Saunders.)

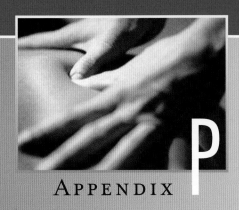

P

STRUCTURES OF THE BODY

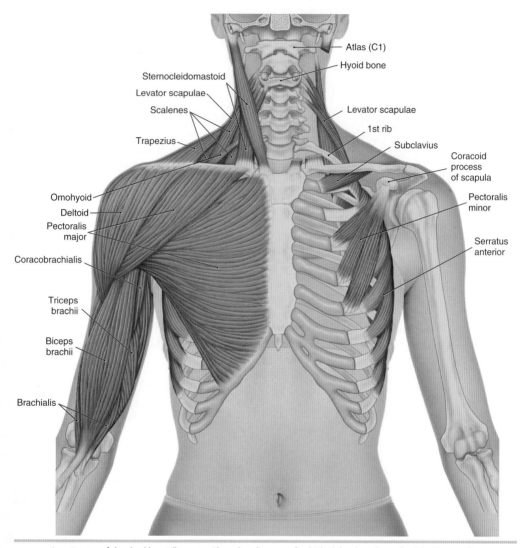

Atlas (C1)
Hyoid bone
Sternocleidomastoid
Levator scapulae
Scalenes
Levator scapulae
1st rib
Trapezius
Subclavius
Coracoid process of scapula
Omohyoid
Deltoid
Pectoralis minor
Pectoralis major
Coracobrachialis
Serratus anterior
Triceps brachii
Biceps brachii
Brachialis

P-1 ■ Anterior view of the shoulder girdle region. The right side is superficial. The left side is deep (the deltoid, pectoralis major, trapezius, scalene, omohyoid, and muscles of the arm have been removed; the sternocleidomastoid has been cut). (From Muscolino JE: *The muscle and bone palpation manual with trigger points, referral patterns and stretching,* St Louis, 2009, Mosby.)

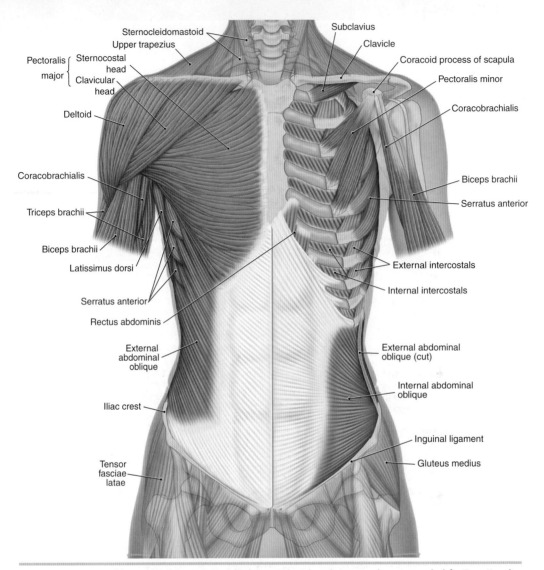

P-2 ■ Anterior view of the muscles of the trunk. Superficial view on the right and an intermediate view on the left. (From Muscolino JE: *The muscle and bone palpation manual with trigger points, referral patterns and stretching,* St Louis, 2009, Mosby.)

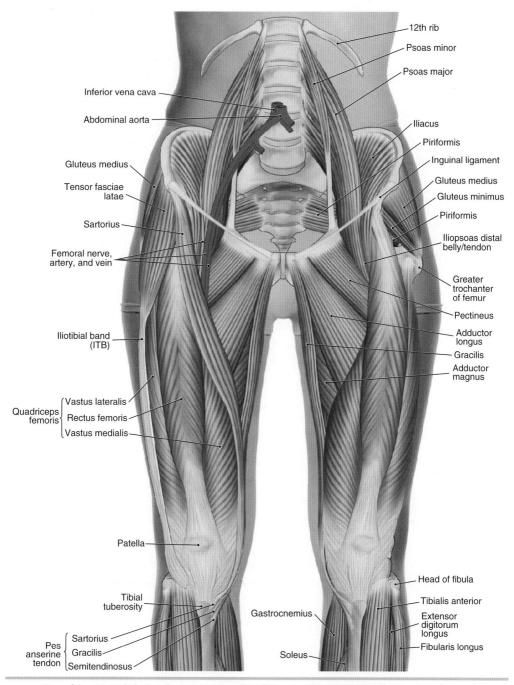

P-3 ■ View of the anterior thigh. Superficial view on the right and an intermediate view on the left. (From Muscolino JE: *The muscle and bone palpation manual with trigger points, referral patterns and stretching,* St Louis, 2009, Mosby.)

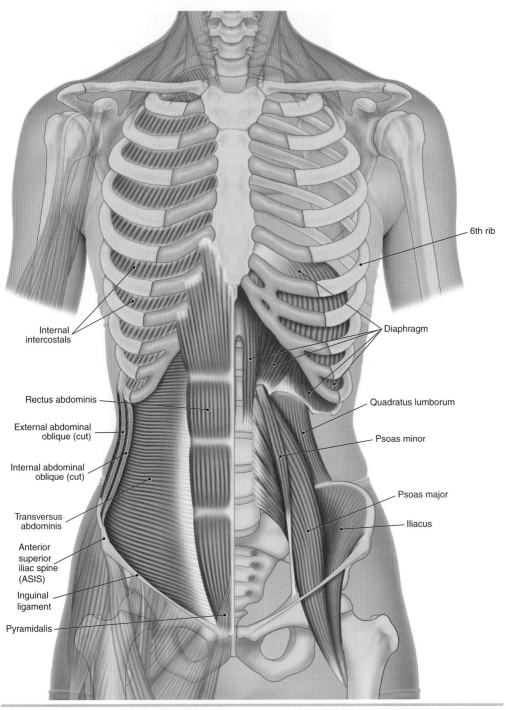

P-4 ▦ Deeper views with the posterior abdominal wall seen on the left. (From Muscolino JE: *The muscle and bone palpation manual with trigger points, referral patterns and stretching,* St, Louis, 2009, Mosby.)

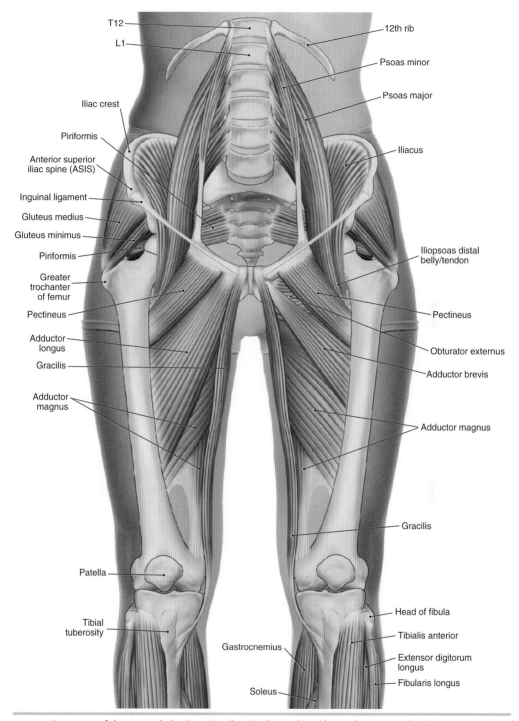

T12

L1

12th rib

Psoas minor

Psoas major

Iliac crest

Piriformis

Iliacus

Anterior superior
iliac spine (ASIS)

Inguinal ligament

Gluteus medius

Gluteus minimus

Piriformis

Iliopsoas distal
belly/tendon

Greater
trochanter
of femur

Pectineus

Pectineus

Adductor
longus

Gracilis

Obturator externus

Adductor brevis

Adductor
magnus

Adductor magnus

Gracilis

Patella

Tibial
tuberosity

Head of fibula

Tibialis anterior

Gastrocnemius

Extensor digitorum
longus

Fibularis longus

Soleus

P-5 ■ Deeper view of the anterior thigh. (From Muscolino JE: *The muscle and bone palpation manual with trigger points, referral patterns and stretching*, St Louis, 2009, Mosby.)

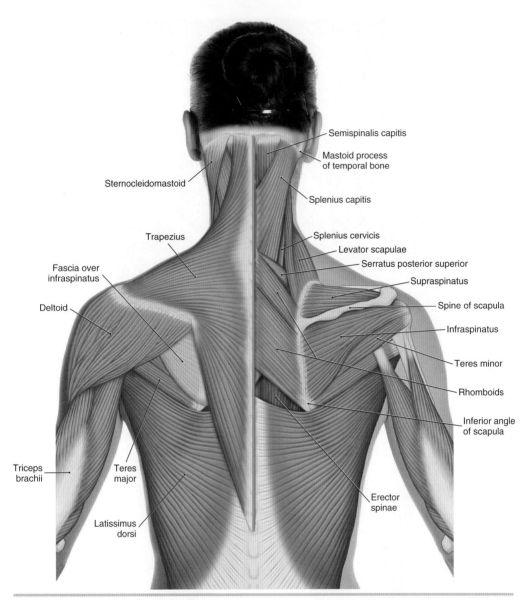

P-6 ■ Posterior view of the shoulder girdle region. The left side is superficial. The right side is deep (the deltoid, trapezius, sternocleidomastoid, and infraspinatus fascia have been removed). (From Muscolino JE: *The muscle and bone palpation manual with trigger points, referral patterns and stretching,* St Louis, 2009, Mosby.)

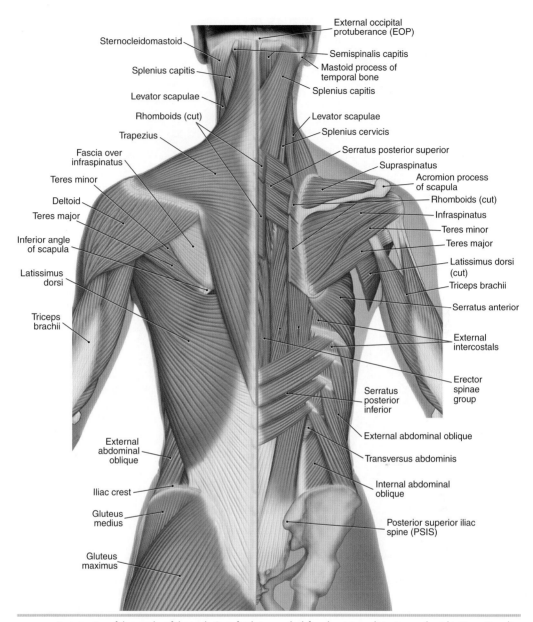

P-7 ▦ Posterior view of the muscles of the trunk. Superficial view on the left and an intermediate view on the right. (From Muscolino JE: *The muscle and bone palpation manual with trigger points, referral patterns and stretching*, St Louis, 2009, Mosby.)

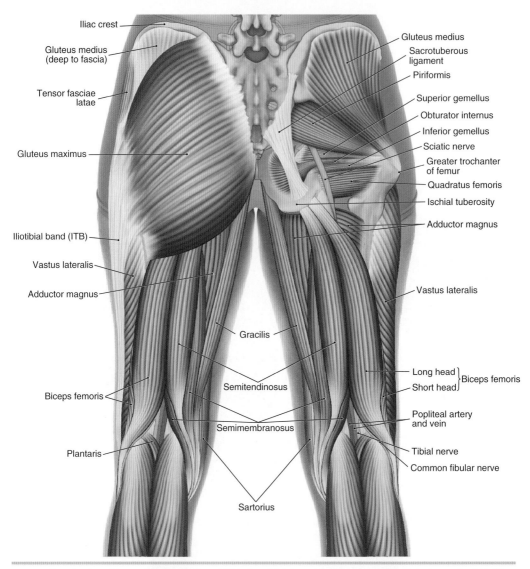

P-8 ■ Posterior view of the muscles of the pelvis and thigh. Superficial view on the left and an intermediate view on the right. (From Muscolino JE: *The muscle and bone palpation manual with trigger points, referral patterns and stretching,* St Louis, 2009, Mosby.)

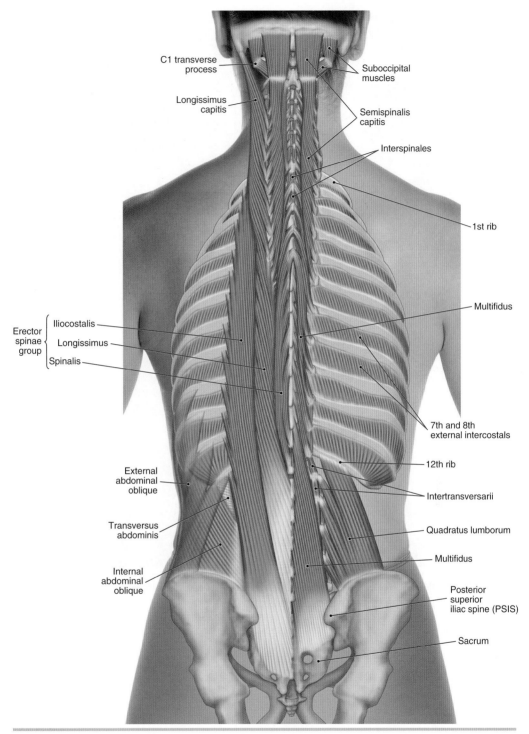

C1 transverse
process

Longissimus
capitis

Suboccipital
muscles

Semispinalis
capitis

Interspinales

1st rib

Multifidus

Erector
spinae
group
— Iliocostalis

— Longissimus

— Spinalis

7th and 8th
external intercostals

External
abdominal
oblique

12th rib

Intertransversarii

Transversus
abdominis

Quadratus lumborum

Internal
abdominal
oblique

Multifidus

Posterior
superior
iliac spine (PSIS)

Sacrum

P-9 ■ Two deeper views of the posterior trunk, the right side deeper than the left. (From Muscolino JE: *The muscle and bone palpation manual with trigger points, referral patterns and stretching,* St Louis, 2009, Mosby.)

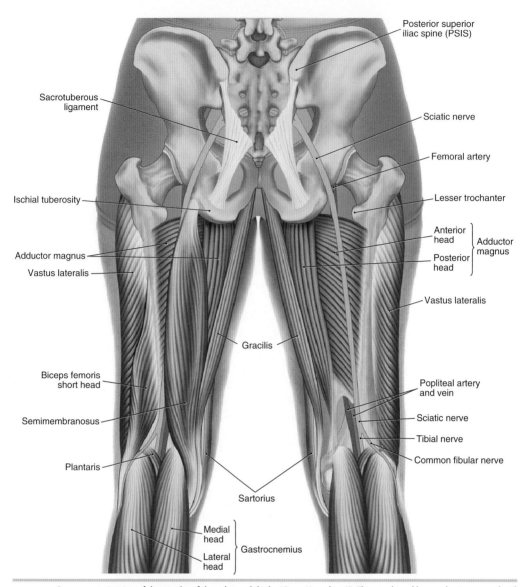

P-10 ■ Deeper posterior view of the muscles of the pelvis and thigh. (*From Muscolino JE: The muscle and bone palpation manual with trigger points, referral patterns and stretching,* St Louis, 2009, Mosby.)

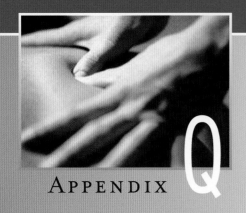

APPENDIX Q

TRIGGER POINTS AND REFERRAL PATTERNS

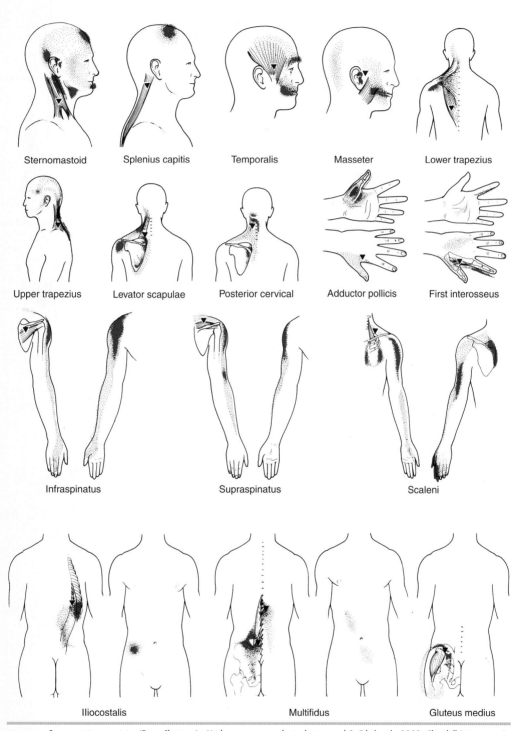

Sternomastoid

Splenius capitis

Temporalis

Masseter

Lower trapezius

Upper trapezius

Levator scapulae

Posterior cervical

Adductor pollicis

First interosseus

Infraspinatus

Supraspinatus

Scaleni

Iliocostalis

Multifidus

Gluteus medius

Q-I ▓ Common trigger points. (From Chaitow L: *Modern neuromuscular techniques,* ed 2, Edinburgh, 2003, Churchill Livingstone.)

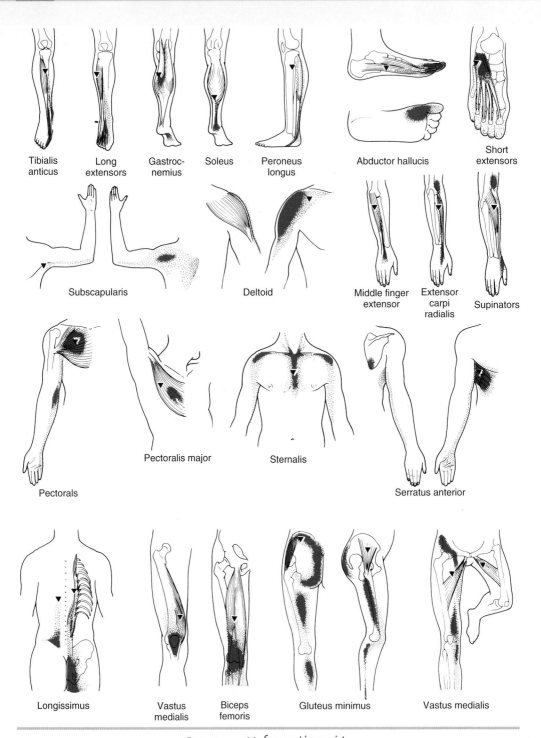

Q-I ■ cont'd. Common trigger points.

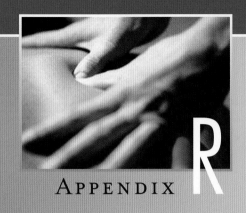

APPENDIX R

ENDANGERMENT SITES

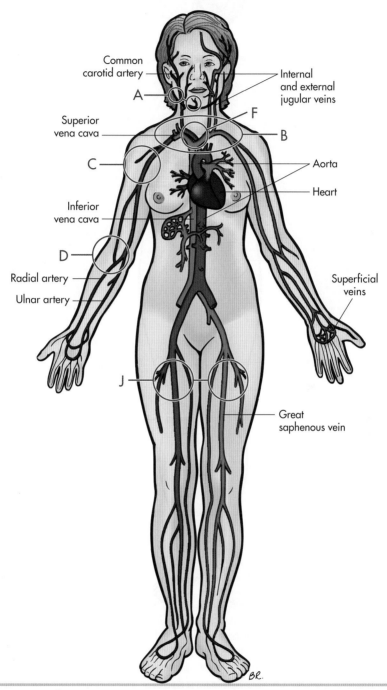

Common
carotid artery

Internal
and external
jugular veins

A

F

Superior
vena cava

B

C

Aorta

Heart

Inferior
vena cava

D

Radial artery

Superficial
veins

Ulnar artery

J

Great
saphenous vein

BR.

R-1 ▥ Endangerment sites of the nervous system and the cardiovascular system. **A,** Anterior triangle of the neck—carotid artery, jugular vein, and vagus nerve, which are located deep to the sternocleidomastoid muscle. **B,** Posterior triangle of the neck—specifically the nerves of the brachial plexus, the brachiocephalic artery and vein superior to the clavicle, and the subclavian arteries and vein. **C,** Axillary area—the brachial artery, axillary vein and artery, cephalic vein, and nerves of the brachial plexus. **D,** Medial epicondyle of the humerus—the ulnar nerve; also the radial and ulnar arteries. **E,** Lateral epicondyle—the radial nerve. **F,** Area of the sterna notch and anterior throat—nerves

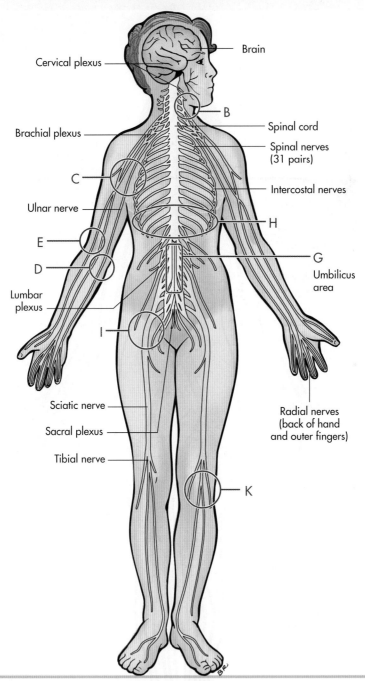

Brain

Cervical plexus

B

Spinal cord

Brachial plexus

Spinal nerves
(31 pairs)

C

Intercostal nerves

Ulnar nerve

H

E

G

D

Umbilicus
area

Lumbar
plexus

I

Sciatic nerve

Radial nerves
(back of hand
and outer fingers)

Sacral plexus

Tibial nerve

K

R-1 ▦ cont'd. and vessels to the thyroid gland and the vagus nerve. **G,** Umbilicus area — to either side; descending aorta and abdominal aorta. **H,** Twelfth rib, dorsal body — location of the kidney. **I,** Sciatic notch — sciatic nerve (the sciatic nerve passes out of the pelvis through the greater sciatic foramen, under cover of the piriformis muscle). **J,** Inguinal triangle located lateral and inferior to the pubis — medial to the sartorius, external iliac artery, femoral artery, great saphenous vein, femoral vein, and femoral nerve. **K,** Popliteal fossa — popliteal artery and vein and tibial nerve. (From Fritz S: *Mosby's fundamentals of therapeutic massage,* ed 4, St Louis, 2009, Mosby.)

GLOSSARY

acetabulum: The concave surface of the pelvis where the femur attaches. The pelvic portion of the hip joint.

acromioclavicular joint: The joint where the acromion process of the scapula and the clavicle meet.

acromioclavicular joint injury grades: Levels of injury to describe joint injuries; grade I is minor tearing with less than 4 mm separation, grade II is moderate tearing with dislocation of the joint, and grade III is complete tearing or rupture of both ligaments and dislocation of the acromioclavicular joint.

acute compartment syndrome: A type of compartment syndrome caused by trauma such as an injury sustained in a car accident. This increases the pressure inside the compartments of the lower leg to the point at which it interferes with the blood supply to the structures. This is a severe injury and should be treated as a medical emergency.

adhesive capsulitis: A disorder in which the shoulder capsule—the connective tissue surrounding the glenohumeral joint of the shoulder—becomes inflamed and stiff, greatly restricting motion and causing chronic pain. This disorder is also known as *frozen shoulder*.

annular ligament: The ligament that wraps around the head of the radius, holding it in place to the ulna at the elbow.

anterior tilt (anterior pelvic rotation): Anterior movement of the upper pelvis; the iliac crest tilts forward in a sagittal plane.

assessment: The collection and interpretation of information provided by the client, the client's family and friends, the massage practitioner, and referring medical professionals. This information includes health history, visual and manual assessments, posture, range of motion, pain levels, and so on.

atlas (C1): The first cervical vertebrae of the spinal column.

axial skeleton: The axis of the body; the axial skeleton consists of the head, vertebral column, ribs, and sternum.

axillary nerve: A branch of the brachial plexus originating from nerves C5 and C6, which carries motor impulses to the shoulder and sensory information from the shoulder joint.

axis (C2): The second cervical vertebrae of the spinal column.

ballistic stretching: A form of stretching involving dynamic or bouncing motions to force the limb into an extended range of motion.

bend: Bending forces are a result of compression and tension combined in one action. Bending involves an external force that is applied perpendicular to the axis of the object. Much like torsion, a compressive force is applied to one side of the object while the other side is exposed to tensile forces.

body alignment: Reference to how the body, bones, joints, and tissues are positioned at a specific point in time or activity.

body mechanics: Use of the body in an efficient and biomechanically correct way.

body positioning: The position of the body in time and space.

borders: A boundary or edge of a surface or area. Used to describe physical edges of a particular object.

brachial plexus: Division of the peripheral nervous system originating from spinal nerves C5-T1, providing sensory and motor function to the shoulder, arms, and hands.

carotid artery: The artery that branches off the arch of the aorta to supply oxygenated blood to the neck and head.

carpal tunnel: An anatomic structure in the wrist formed by the carpal bones and the transverse carpal ligament.

carpal tunnel syndrome: A disorder in which the median nerve is compressed at the wrist in the carpal tunnel, creating numbness, tingling, pain, and weakness in the first three digits and half of the fourth digit.

central nervous system: The division of the nervous system consisting of the brain, brain stem, and spinal cord.

cervical plexus: The group of spinal nerves C1-C4 that innervate the posterior neck and head.

cervical vertebrae: A group of seven vertebrae found just inferior to the skull and form the neck.

chronic compartment syndrome: An exercise-induced disorder in which the pressure within anatomic compartments increases, resulting in compromised circulation and function of the tissues in the compartment. This disorder is recurrent and results in pain and discomfort, which subsides when activity is stopped.

closed chain: The positioning of joints in such a way that motion at one of the joints is accompanied by motion at an adjacent joint.

compartment syndrome: A disorder in which the pressure within closed anatomic spaces increases, resulting in compromised circulation and functions of the tissues in the compartment. This can be a serious and life-threatening disorder.

compartments of the leg: The lower leg has four compartments divided by the interosseous membrane, transverse intermuscular septum, and posterior intermuscular septum. These compartments are the anterior, lateral, deep posterior, and superficial posterior compartments.

compensation pattern: The process of counterbalancing a defect in body structure or function. These counterbalancing actions can be predicted and result in specific patterns throughout the body.

compression: Pressure into the body to compress tissues against underlying structures. (This massage manipulation sometimes is classified with pétrissage.) Also, the exertion of inappropriate pressure on nerves by hard tissue (e.g., bone).

congenital torticollis: Torticollis that presents itself at birth or shortly after birth.

connective tissue massage: A modality of massage that focuses on the connective tissues of the body. This modality can include, but is not limited to, techniques such as Bindegewebs massage, myofascial massage techniques, deep tissue, Rolfing, and Hellerwork.

deep lateral rotators or deep six muscles: A group of muscles that work together to cause lateral rotation of the hip. These muscles include the piriformis, gemellus superior, gemellus inferior, obturator internus, obturator externus, and quadratus femoris.

deep layer: A layer of tissues located deep or further from the surface within a specific area.

deep tissue massage: Deep tissue massage focuses on addressing the muscular complaints that are rooted in the deeper layers of the musculoskeletal system. Deep tissue massage should not be viewed as a separate modality, but rather as a use of several different techniques of therapeutic massage to enhance the overall outcome of the session. Deep tissue massage is a mindset, an intention, and an approach to address specific musculoskeletal complaints.

deepest layer: The layer of tissues found deepest in the body. Usually used to describe the fascia found in the craniosacral system or the visceral fascia.

depth of pressure: Compressive forces that can be light, moderate, deep, or varied.

distal radioulnar joint: The articulation between the radius and ulna located near the wrist.

distal ulnar tunnel (Guyon canal): The tunnel through which the ulnar nerve passes at the wrist. It is formed by the ulnar and carpal bones, the pisohamate ligament, the palmar carpal ligament, and the transverse carpal ligament.

dynamic stretching: A form of stretching that uses momentum to take the muscle into an extended range of motion, not exceeding the person's static-passive range of motion.

edema: The accumulation of abnormal amounts of fluid in the interstitial spaces. There are different types of edema such as pitting, skin, generalized, peripheral, and pulmonary.

effleurage: Gliding, horizontal strokes applied with the fingers, hand, or forearm that usually follow the fiber direction of the underlying muscle, fascial planes, or dermatome pattern.

ergonomics: The applied science of workplace, equipment, and design factors intended to maximize productivity and reduce fatigue and discomfort.

exertional or tension headache: The most common form of headache caused by stress, tension, tight muscles, inadequate rest, poor posture, anxiety, or fatigue.

external rotators: A group of muscles that cause rotation away from the midline at a specific joint. Often referred to as the *lateral rotators*.

fascia: A fibrous or loose type of connective tissue; a fibrous membrane covering, supporting, and separating muscles; the subcutaneous tissue that connects the skin to the muscles.

fibrous joint capsule: An articular capsule composed of white fibrous tissue, which surrounds a synovial joint connecting bone to bone.

flattening of the spine: A descriptive term often used to describe a decrease in the natural curvature of the spine.

forward head: A descriptive term used to describe a common postural disorder in which the head is in a position forward of the center of the shoulders, resulting in a hyperlordotic curvature of the upper cervical vertebrae and hypolordotic curvature of the lower cervical vertebrae.

friction: Specific circular or transverse movements that do not glide on the skin and that are focused on the underlying tissue.

functional anatomy: The study of anatomy specific to its function.

functional scoliosis: Scoliosis that is not caused by a structural bone disorder. Functional scoliosis is a temporary disorder caused by functional or postural distortions such as a leg length difference, hypertonic muscles, or an inflammatory condition.

gait assessment: The observation and analysis of the way a person walks.

glenohumeral joint: The ball-and-socket joint located in the shoulder where the humerus and scapula meet.

grades of sprains and strains: A system to describe the severity of muscular strains and ligamental sprains. There are three grades: grade 1 is minor tearing, grade 2 is moderate tearing, and grade 3 is severe tearing or complete rupture.

gravitational forces: Push or pull on an object in an attempt to affect motion or shape. The pull of an object towards the Earth, or gravity and its affects on the body in a static position or during movement.

gross anatomy: The study of body structures visible to the naked eye.

gross movements: Involves large muscles and multiple muscles used to create major movements like walking, running, sitting, and other movements.

headache (HA): A disorder that creates pain in the head often caused by muscular tension, stress, hormone, circulation, or other disturbance. Common types of headaches include migraine, sinus, tension, cluster, and hormonal.

heel spur: A bony growth or projection on the posterior or plantar surface of the calcaneus bone.

Hellerwork: A form of massage therapy focused on the deep connective tissues of the body. Often referred to as *structural bodywork*. Hellerwork focuses on the vertical alignment of the body and release of chronic stress and tension.

homeostasis: The relatively constant state of the internal environment of the body that is maintained by adaptive responses. Specific control and feedback mechanisms are responsible for adjusting body systems to maintain this state.

humeroradial joint: The articulation between the humerus bone and the head of the radius located in the elbow.

humeroulnar joint: The articulation between the humerus bone and the ulna bone located in the elbow.

hyperkyphosis: An increased convex curvature of the thoracic curvature of the spine.

hyperlordosis: An increased forward curvature of the cervical or lumbar spine.

hypertonicity: An area of increased tone or tension. Often used to describe muscular or arterial tension.

hypokyphosis: A decrease in the natural convex curvature of the thoracic spine.

hypolordosis: A decrease in the natural curvature of the cervical or lumbar spine.

iliotibial band disorder: A condition of the lateral thigh and knee often caused by friction of the fascia band over the lateral epicondyle of the femur. Activities like running, hiking, weight training, or cycling can cause and aggravate this disorder, resulting in knee pain.

iliotibial (IT) band or tract: The thick band of fascia that runs from the gluteus maximus and the tensor fascia latae to Gerdy tubercle at the lateral surface of the tibia.

impingement: Pressure against a structure by skin, fascia, muscles, ligaments, or joints.

intention: The act of intending, or to act in a certain way. The course a person aims to follow.

internal rotators: A group of muscles that work together to create internal or medial rotation at a joint.

interphalangeal (IP) joint: the joint located between two phalanges. The phalanges may have a distal interphalangeal joint or a proximal interphalangeal joint.

ischemia: A deficiency or decreased supply of blood to a tissue.

joint movements: The movements of the joint through its normal range of motion.

jugular vein: The vein that carries blood from the head back to the heart.

kinematics: A branch of mechanics that involves the aspects of time, space, and mass in a moving system.

kinesiology: The study of movement that combines the fields of anatomy, physiology, physics, and geometry, and relates them to human movement.

kinetic chain: The process by which each individual joint movement pattern is part of an interconnected aspect of the neurologic coordination pattern of muscle movement.

kyphosis: A condition of exaggeration of the thoracic curve.

lateral collateral ligament: A ligament located on the outside of a joint. Also known as the *radial ligament* in the elbow or the *fibular ligament* in the knee.

layer: A layer of muscles that overlies or underlies another layer. It is used to describe the location within the body.

locomotion: Moving from one place to another; walking.

lordosis: A condition of exaggeration of the normal lumbar curve.

lower crossed syndrome: A syndrome that describes tight and weak muscles that develops because of postural habits in the pelvic region.

massage modalities: A specific approach or technique used in massage.

mechanical forces: Forces applied to create an anatomic or physiologic change in the body. These forces can include actions such as pushing, pulling, or friction. The five common mechanical forces are compression, tension, bending, torsion, and shear.

medial collateral ligament: A ligament located on the inside or medial surface of a joint. Also known as the *ulnar ligament* in the elbow or the *tibial ligament* in the knee.

median nerve: A nerve branching from the brachial plexus (C6-C8) that innervates the forearm flexors, palmar surface, and digits 1–3 and half of digit 4.

metacarpophalangeal (MCP) joint: Joint located between the metacarpals and the phalanges of the hand.

micromovements: Small movements that take place within the body anatomically and physiologically.

microtears: Small or tiny tears found in tendons, muscles, or ligaments.

microtrauma: General term given to small, often unnoticed injuries to the body often caused by overuse or repetitive stress.

migraine: A severe form of a headache characterized by intense throbbing in one area of the head. Often accompanied by vomiting, nausea, and sensitivity to light and sound. This form of headache can be debilitating.

muscle belly: The portion of the muscle where the muscle fibers are found. This is the region between the tendons.

muscle strain: An injury to the muscle in which the muscles fibers tear as a result of trauma or overstretching.

muscular layers: Term used to describe the muscles in reference to the depth of the tissues.

musculocutaneous nerve: Branch of the brachial plexus from nerves C5-C7 that innervates the bicep brachialis, coracobrachialis, and the brachialis.

musculotendinous junction: The point where muscle fibers end and the connective tissue continues to form the tendon; a major site of injury.

musculotendinous: Refers to the area where the muscle and tendon merge.

myofascial massage: Styles of bodywork that affect the connective tissues; often called *deep tissue massage, soft tissue manipulation,* or *myofascial release.*

myofascial release: A system of bodywork that affects the connective tissue of the body through various methods that elongate and alter the plastic component and ground matrix of the connective tissue.

neutral position: The position where minimal stress is placed on the joint, bone, or muscle.

nonverbal signs: A form of feedback where oral communication is not taking place. These signs can include body twitches, changes in position, respiration, changes in skin temperature, or facial expression.

normal posture: The postural alignment in which the client spends most of his or her time. This refers to the way a person is standing or sitting at rest.

objective: A goal or outcome. It is also the section of SOAP notes in which the therapist writes out all observations he or she notices.

open chains: A position in which the ends of the limbs or parts of the body are free to move without causing motion at another joint.

organic headache: A general headache or pain in the head resulting from a change in the organ systems of the body (i.e. hormonal or circulatory).

PRICE principle: Protection, rest, ice, compression, elevation.

pain-spasm-pain cycle: Steady contraction of muscles, which causes ischemia and stimulates pain receptors in muscles. The pain, in turn, initiates more spasms, which trigger a self-sustaining injury.

patellofemoral dysfunction: A disorder in which there is an increase in pressure and friction between the patella and femur, resulting in generalized knee pain.

pelvis: The region of the skeleton consisting of the ilium, ischium, and pubis.

periostitis: Inflammation of the fascial membrane that surrounds the bone.

periosteum: The dense connective tissue that envelops the bones.

peripheral nervous system: The system of somatic and autonomic neurons outside the central nervous system. The peripheral nervous system comprises the afferent (sensory) division and the efferent (motor) division.

pétrissage: Kneading: rhythmic rolling, lifting, squeezing, and wringing of soft tissue.

physiology: The study of the processes and functions of the body involved in supporting life.

plan: The portion of the SOAP notes in which the client and therapist write the long-term and short-term goals of their sessions and the process to achieve these goals.

plantar fascia: The thick connective tissue found on the plantar surface of the foot, which supports the arch of the foot.

plantar fasciitis: Inflammation of the plantar fascia.

posterior tilt: Posterior movement of the upper pelvis in which the iliac crest tilts and the pubis moves superiorly. Often a result of tight lateral rotators of the hips, hamstrings, and abdominal muscles.

postisometric relaxation (PIR): The state that occurs after isometric contraction of a muscle; it results from the activity of minute neural reporting stations called the Golgi Tendon Organs.

postural assessment: The process of evaluating a personal position to determine symmetry and balance in relation to anatomically correct posture.

postural distortions: Deviations from the anatomically correct posture.

postural muscles: Muscles that support the body against gravity.

postural patterning: The patterns created by habitual positioning and movement, which may result in deviations or restricted muscles in the body.

posture: The position of the body when standing or sitting.

primary: The first or highest in a rank, quality, or importance.

principles of deep tissue massage: The fundamental rules of deep tissue massage.

pronator teres syndrome: A disorder that results in the compression of the median nerve at the elbow.

proximal radioulnar joint: The joint where the radial head articulates with the ulna at the elbow.

proximal ulnar (cubital) tunnel: The channel through which the ulnar nerve travels at the elbow.

radial nerve: A branch from the brachial plexus that innervates the triceps, forearm extensors, and hand.

range of motion for the cervical vertebrae: The amount of movement available at the neck.

repetitive motions: Movements or actions that are repeated often and for long periods.

Rolfing: A form of deep connective tissue massage developed by Ida Rolf and often referred to as *structural bodywork*.

rotator cuff: The group of muscles and their tendons that act to stabilize the shoulder. Often used to refer to the SITS muscles: supraspinatus, infraspinatus, teres minor, and subscapularis.

sciatica: A disorder in which there is an increase in pressure on the sciatic nerve causing pain, weakness, numbness, or tingling in the leg.

scoliosis: A lateral curvature of the spine.

secondary: Coming after, or next in line of importance. The second in rank of importance.

shear: A shear force occurs when two structures slide across each other and create friction.

shin splints: A general term used to describe pain in the lower anterior leg. Also known as *tibial stress syndrome.* Shin splints are a result of muscular stress or trauma.

shoulder girdle: The bones that support the upper limb. Refers to the scapula and clavicle.

spasmodic torticollis: Also known as *wry-neck,* this is a condition in which the neck muscles contract involuntarily, causing the head to turn or twist to one side.

speed: Rate of application (i.e., fast, slow, varied).

sprains: A disorder in which the ligaments of a joint tear or rupture.

stability: The state of being stable or balanced.

stages of adhesive capsulitis: The three stages someone with adhesive capsulitis goes through are freezing, frozen, and thawing.

static stretching: Stretching where the body is relaxed, which takes the muscle to a level of gentle tension and is held for several seconds. Often referred to as *passive stretching.*

sternoclavicular joint: The joint that holds the upper extremities to the body. This is where the clavicle and the sternum join.

stress: Any substantial change in routine or any activity that forces the body to adapt.

stressor: Any internal perceptions or external stimuli that demand a change in the body.

structural integration: Method of bodywork derived from biomechanics, postural alignment, and the importance of the connective tissue structures.

structural scoliosis: A lateral or rotating curvature of the spine resulting from bone malformation, connective tissue disorders, or other disease.

subjective: The section of SOAP notes in which information the client shares with the therapist is written.

suboccipital: The area located under or below the occipital bone.

superficial: Referring to the surface or outer area.

superficial layer: The layer that is outermost or at the surface of the body.

tapotement: Repetitive blows to the body using the palms, fists, fingers, or edge of the hands in a rhythmic pattern to compress the tissue; also called *percussion.*

temporomandibular joint (TMJ): The joint in the head where the mandible and temporal bone join.

tendon: A band of connective tissue that connects muscles to bone.

tendonitis: Inflammation of the tendon often caused by overuse.

tendinosis: A degeneration of the tendon caused by damage to the tendon at a cellular level.

tensile force: A pulling force, the opposite of compression.

tension: A tensile force in which the ends of the object are being pulled in the opposite direction from each other.

tensor fascia latae: The muscle located in the lateral hip that connects the iliac crest to the iliotibial band or tract

thixotropy: The property of becoming less viscous when moved or shaken.

thoracic outlet syndrome (TOS): A group of disorders that occurs when the blood vessels and nerves in the thoracic outlet become compressed.

thoracolumbar fascia: The thick fascial band located on the posterior surface of the body that covers the muscles of the low back.

thoracopelvic region: The region of the body referring to the chest, abdomen, and pelvis.

thorax: Also known as the *chest cavity.* The thorax is the upper region of the torso. It is enclosed by the sternum, ribs, and thoracic vertebrae and contains the lungs, heart, and great blood vessels.

tibial stress syndrome: A general term used to describe pain in the lower anterior leg caused by muscular stress or trauma. Also known as *shin splints.*

torsion: Torsion is the application of a twisting or turning force to an object. This twisting force most often involves one direction at one end of an object and is stabilized or moved in the opposite direction at the other end. During this movement both tensile and compressive forces are acting on a specific area at the same time.

touch without movement: Contact with no movement.

toxic headache: Headache resulting from exposure to toxic substances, fever, or bacterial infection.

traction and distraction: Gentle pull on the joint capsule to increase the joint space.

transverse carpal ligament (flexor retinaculum): The dense connective tissue located in the wrist between the hamate and pisiform bones to the scaphoid and trapezium bones.

trigger point: A hyperirritable locus within a taut band of skeletal muscle, located in the muscular tissue or its associated fascia. The spot is painful on compression and can evoke characteristic referred pain and autonomic phenomena.

tunnel: A covered passageway.

ulnar nerve: The nerve branch from the brachial plexus that innervates the muscles of the hand and the skin of digits 4 and 5.

upper crossed syndrome: A pattern of tight and weak muscles that creates a postural distortion in the upper body as a result of habitual postural patterns.

verbal signs: Oral communications or feedback between the client and therapist.

vibration: Fine or coarse tremulous movement that creates reflexive responses.

whiplash: An injury to the soft tissues of the neck caused by sudden hyperextension or flexion of the neck.

winged scapula: A condition in which the scapula protrudes from a person's back.

withdrawing: To pull out of or to take away from a particular place.

Wolff's law: Law of bone adaptation. States that bone in a healthy person will adapt to the load that is placed on it. If the load increases, bone will remodel itself to become stronger. If it is lessened, the bone will become weaker.

REFERENCES

Books

Anderson B: *Stretching*, Bolinas, 1980, Shelter Publications.

Armiger P, Martyn M: *Stretching for functional flexibility*, Baltimore, 2010, Lippincott, Williams & Wilkins.

Barnes JF: *Myofascial release: the search for excellence*, Paoli, 1990, John F. Barnes, P.T.

Beck M: *Theory and practice of therapeutic massage*, ed 4, Clifton Park, 2006, Cengage.

Benjamin P: *Tappan's handbook of healing massage techniques*, ed 5, Upper Saddle River, 2010, Pearson.

Biel A: *Trail guide to the body*, ed 3, Boulder, 2005, Books of Discovery.

Braun MB, Simonson S: *Introduction to massage therapy*, Baltimore, 2008, Lippincott, Williams & Wilkins.

Burman I, Friedland S: *TouchAbilities: essential connections*, Clifton Park, 2006, Cengage.

Chaitow L: *Palpation and assessment skills*, ed 2, St. Louis, 2006, Churchill Livingstone.

Chaitow L, Fritz S: *A massage therapist's guide to understanding, locating and treating myofascial trigger points*, St. Louis, 2006, Churchill Livingstone.

Clay J, Pounds D: *Basic clinical massage therapy; integrating anatomy and treatment*, ed 2, Baltimore, 2008, Lippincott, Williams & Wilkins.

Dalton E: *Erik Dalton's advanced myoskeletal techniques*, Oklahoma City, 2005, Freedom from Pain Institute.

Dorland's pocket medical dictionary, ed 28, St. Louis, 2009, Saunders.

Ebrall P: *Assessment of the spine*, St. Louis, 2004, Churchill Livingstone.

Fernandez F: *Deep tissue massage treatment: a handbook of neuromuscular therapy*, St. Louis, 2006, Mosby.

Field D: *Anatomy palpation and surface markings*, ed 3, St. Louis, 2005, Elsevier.

Fritz S, Grosenback MJ: *Mosby's essential sciences for therapeutic massage*, ed 3, St. Louis, 2009, Mosby.

Fritz S: *Mosby's fundamentals of therapeutic massage*, ed 4, St. Louis, 2009, Mosby.

Hendrickson T: *Massage and manual therapy for orthopedic conditions*, ed 2, Baltimore, 2009, Lippincott, Williams & Wilkins.

Hoppenfeld S: *Physical examination of the spine and extremities*, Upper Saddle River, 1976, Prentice-Hall.

Johnson J: *Deep tissue massage*, Champaign, 2010, Human Kinetics.

Kendall F, McCreary E, Provance P, et al: *Muscles: testing and function with posture and pain*, ed 5, Baltimore, 2005, Lippincott, Williams & Wilkins.

Lowe W: *Orthopedic assessment in massage therapy*, Sisters, 2006, Daviau Scott Publishers.

Magee D: *Orthopedic physical assessment*, ed 5, St. Louis, 2008, Saunders.

McAtee RE: *Facilitated stretching*, Champaign, 1993, Human Kinetics.

Muscolino JE: *Kinesiology: the skeletal system and muscle function*, St. Louis, 2006, Mosby.

Muscolino JE: *The muscle and bone palpation manual with trigger points, referral patterns, and stretching*, St. Louis, 2009, Mosby.

Muscolino J: *The muscular system manual*, St. Louis, 2009, Mosby.

Myers T: *Anatomy trains: myofascial meridians for manual movement therapists*, St. Louis, 2001, Churchill Livingstone.

Oatis C: *Kinesiology: the mechanics and pathomechanics of human movement*, ed 2, Baltimore, 2009, Lippincott, Williams & Wilkins.

Riggs A: *Deep tissue massage: a visual guide to techniques*, Berkley, 2007, North Atlantic Books.

Salvo SG: *Massage therapy: principles and practice*, ed 3, St. Louis, 2007, Saunders.

Scheumann D: *The balance body: a guide to deep tissue and neuromuscular therapy*, ed 3, Baltimore, 2007, Lippincott, Williams & Wilkins.

Smith J: *Structural bodywork: an introduction for students and practitioners*, St. Louis, 2005, Churchill Livingstone.

Stanborough M: *Direct release myofascial technique an illustrated guide for practitioners*, St. Louis, 2004, Churchill Livingstone.

Stillerman E: *Modalities for massage and bodywork*, ed 1, St. Louis, 2009, Elsevier.

Turchaninov R: *Therapeutic massage: a scientific approach*, Phoenix, 2000, Aesculapius Books.

Turchaninov R: *Medical massage*, ed 2, Phoenix, 2006, Aesculapius Books.

Werner R: *A massage therapist's guide to pathology*, ed 4, Baltimore, 2009, Lippincott, Williams, & Wilkins.

Websites

Connective Tissue Massage (CTM) Bindegewebs Massage Website: http://www.ctm-bindegewebsmassage.com/.
European Rolfing Association: http://www.rolfing.org.
Freedom from Pain Institute Website: http://ericdalton.com.
Learnmuscles.com: *The Art and Science of Kinesiology.* http://learnmuscles.com.
Massage and Bodywork Magazine: http://www.massageandbodywork.com.
Massagetherapy.com: http://www.massagetherapy.com.
MTJ: Massage Therapy Journal: http://www.amtamassage.org/articles/3/mtj/index.html.
Rolf Institute of Structural Integration: http://www.rolf.org.

Journals

Riggs A: Deep tissue massage part 1: the tools, *Massage & Bodywork* 38–46, February/March 2005.
Riggs A: Deep tissue massage part 2: stroke intention, *Massage & Bodywork* 60–69, April/May 2005.
Riggs A: Deep tissue massage part 3: body position, *Massage & Bodywork* 72–80, June/July 2005.
Riggs A: Deep, but not too deep, *Massage & Bodywork* 32–33, July/August 2010.

INDEX

Note: Page numbers followed by *f* indicate figures; *t*, table; *b*, boxes.